Solving Critical Consults

Core Principles of Acute Neurology:

Recognizing Brain Injury
Providing Acute Care
Handling Difficult Situations
Communicating Prognosis
Identifying Neuroemergencies

Solving Critical Consults

EELCO F. M. WIJDICKS, M.D., PH.D., FACP, FNCS, FANA
Professor of Neurology, Mayo College of Medicine
Chair, Division of Critical Care Neurology
Consultant, Neurosciences Intensive Care Unit
Saint Marys Hospital
Mayo Clinic, Rochester, Minnesota

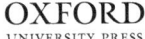

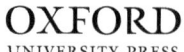
OXFORD
UNIVERSITY PRESS

Oxford University Press is a department of the University of
Oxford. It furthers the University's objective of excellence in research,
scholarship, and education by publishing worldwide.

Oxford New York
Auckland Cape Town Dar es Salaam Hong Kong Karachi
Kuala Lumpur Madrid Melbourne Mexico City Nairobi
New Delhi Shanghai Taipei Toronto

With offices in
Argentina Austria Brazil Chile Czech Republic France Greece
Guatemala Hungary Italy Japan Poland Portugal Singapore
South Korea Switzerland Thailand Turkey Ukraine Vietnam

Oxford is a registered trademark of Oxford University Press
in the UK and certain other countries.

Published in the United States of America by
Oxford University Press
198 Madison Avenue, New York, NY 10016

© 2016 by Mayo Foundation for Medical Education and Research

All rights reserved. No part of this publication may be reproduced, stored in
a retrieval system, or transmitted, in any form or by any means, without the prior
permission in writing of Oxford University Press, or as expressly permitted by law,
by license, or under terms agreed with the appropriate reproduction rights organization.
Inquiries concerning reproduction outside the scope of the above should be sent to the
Rights Department, Oxford University Press, at the address above.

You must not circulate this work in any other form
and you must impose this same condition on any acquirer.

Library of Congress Cataloging-in-Publication Data
Wijdicks, Eelco F. M., 1954– , author.
Solving critical consults / Eelco F. M. Wijdicks.
p. ; cm. — (Core principles of acute neurology)
Includes bibliographical references and index.
ISBN 978–0–19–025109–3 (alk. paper)
I. Title. II. Series: Core principles of acute neurology.
[DNLM: 1. Nervous System Diseases—therapy. 2. Intensive Care—methods.
3. Intensive Care Units. 4. Postoperative Complications. WL 140]
RC86.8
616.02'8—dc23
2015004000

The science of medicine is a rapidly changing field. As new research and clinical experience broaden
our knowledge, changes in treatment and drug therapy occur. The author and publisher of this
work have checked with sources believed to be reliable in their efforts to provide information that
is accurate, complete, and in accordance with the standards accepted at the time of publication.
However, in light of the possibility of human error or changes in the practice of medicine, neither
the author, nor the publisher, nor any other party who has been involved in the preparation or
publication of this work warrants that the information contained herein is in every respect accurate
or complete. Readers are encouraged to confirm the information contained herein with other
reliable sources and are strongly advised to check the product information sheet provided by the
pharmaceutical company for each drug they plan to administer.

For Barbara, Coen, and Marilou

Contents

Preface ix
Introduction to the Series xi

1. Consulting in the Intensive Care Unit 1
2. Acute Confusion in the Critically Ill 17
3. Encephalopathies of Organ Dysfunction 33
4. The Postoperative Cardiac Patient 47
5. Neurologic Urgencies After Vascular Surgery 61
6. Post–Cardiac Arrest Support and the Brain 77
7. Acquired Weakness in the Intensive Care Unit 93
8. Neurology of Polytrauma 107
9. Neurooncology Emergencies 121
10. Troubleshooting: ICU Neurotoxicology 137

Index 151

Preface

Neurologic consultations for critically ill patients are common and may take time. Often, a neurologist is asked to explain changes in the patient's responsiveness or to confirm and manage an obvious neurologic complication. In some patients, one can quickly sense that the presented problem is a less straightforward situation — or worse. Solving a clinical situation which is difficult to understand or put together may be part of an urgent neurology consult.

Intensive care unit (ICU) consults follow certain patterns, and context and substance have crystallized over the years. For this volume I have chosen the most frequent queries. Neurologists can expect consults for patients who do not fully awaken after critical illness (identified by the all-encompassing term "mental status change") or for assessment of muscle weakness (typically immobility and failure to liberate the patient off the ventilator). A new speech problem or some new perceived limb asymmetry or no movement at all is commonly a reason for a STAT consult. Neurologic complications are major when they involve recurrent seizures, postoperative failure to awaken, or acute disabling neuromuscular disease. Consults in general ICU's are less common than consults on the ward and that leaves the question of whether neurologic complications are sufficiently recognized.

The evaluation and management of neurologic complications in acutely ill hospitalized patients should be part of the core principles of acute neurology, and realistically, is a field which is recognizably different. Some requests for consultation include not only assessment of the neurologic state of a critically ill patient but also assistance with management at all levels. Prognostication in devastating situations or when the critical illness has come under control is a common request. A common misperception is that a serious neurologic complication should limit aggressive care of the very sick patient. In some instances, neurologists do not share this pessimism. Assessment of outcome comes with difficult choices.

There is a core of consult topics. The most urgent consults are selected in this volume, with a focus on pathophysiology, mechanisms, and management. This field requires a special expertise and frequent reassessment of the spectrum of complications. Practical advice is included to literally provide a neurologic helping hand to the general intensivist.

Introduction to the Series

The confrontation with an acutely ill neurologic patient is quite an unsettling situation for physicians, but all will have to master how to manage the patient at presentation, how to shepherd the unstable patient to an intensive care unit, and how to take charge. To do that aptly, knowledge of the principles of management is needed. Books on the clinical practice of acute, emergency, and critical care neurology have appeared, but none have yet treated the fundamentals in depth.

Core Principles of Acute Neurology is a series of short volumes that handles topics not found in sufficient detail elsewhere. They focus precisely on those areas that require a good working knowledge. These are the consequences of acute neurologic diseases, medical care in all its aspects and relatedness with the injured brain, and difficult decisions in complex situations. Because the practice involves devastatingly injured patients, there is a separate volume on prognostication and neuropalliation. Other volumes are planned in the future.

The series has unique features. I contextualize basic science with clinical practice in a readable narrative with a light touch and without wielding the jargon of this field. The 10 chapters in each volume clearly details how things work. It is divided into a description of principles followed by its relevance to practice—keeping it to the bare essentials. There are boxes inserted into the text with quick reminders ("By the Way") and useful percentages carefully researched and vetted for accuracy ("By the Numbers"). Drawings are used to illustrate mechanisms and pathophysiology.

These books cannot cover an entire field, but brevity and economy allows a focus on one topic at a time. Gone are the days of large, doorstop tomes with many words on paper but with little practical value. This series is therefore characterized by simplicity—in a good sense—with acute and critical care neurology at the core, not encyclopedic but representative. I hope it supplements clinical curricula or comprehensive textbooks.

The audience are primarily neurologists and neurointensivists, neurosurgeons, fellows, and residents. Neurointensivists have increased in numbers, and many major institutions have attendings and fellowship programs. However, these books cross disciplines and should also be useful for intensivists, anesthesiologists, emergency physicians, nursing staff, and allied health care professionals in intensive care units and the emergency department. In the end the intent is to write a book that provides a sound reassuring basis to practice well, and that helps with understanding and appreciating the complexities of the care of a patient with an acute neurologic condition.

1

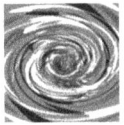

Consulting in the Intensive Care Unit

Teams working in intensive care units (ICUs) may bring in a neurologist, and this happens more frequently as the illness progresses or lingers. There should be no doubt that the complexity of critical illness is astounding for most neurologists entering the ICU. On occasion, multicatheterized patients are surrounded by monitors, stacked infusion pumps, and a dialysis machine, and they may even be supported by an extracorporeal membrane oxygenation device. Nonplussed, neurologists stop for a moment, reluctantly recognizing that the neurologic examination will be truncated, confounded, and less specific than hoped for. The consulting neurologist has to probe deeply into the electronic medical records to find essential information, to check order sets, and to understand the rationale for certain treatment decisions.

The modern ICU is a unique place with unique patients, and consultants have very specific expertise in handling critical illness. Patients come into the ICU already doing very poorly, and when major organs fail and patients become hypotensive, hypoxemic, hypercapnic, or tachycardic, the initial resuscitation typically does not concentrate on neurologic manifestations. Most intensivists briefly check for pupil responses or major asymmetries, but they readily accept that an altered level of consciousness is a common consequence of an evolving critical illness. One can expect that some of the manifestations will be considered not atypical enough to urgently ask for a neurologist.

Critical illness increases the chance of a neurologic complication, and current best estimates are that approximately 5%–10% of patients with critical medical illness will develop some sort of neurologic manifestation.[2,23] Many of these manifestations are transient (e.g., unexplained altered consciousness or brief twitching), but in other cases, there is an acute, evident problem that needs to be emergently addressed.[9,10]

Neurology consultations may include the assessment of coma after cardiopulmonary resuscitation (CPR), assistance with management and evaluation of delirium, exclusion or treatment of seizures, and identification of a previously underlying neuromuscular disorder in a patient who cannot come off the ventilator despite multiple trials.

Most intensivists feel uncomfortable in handling a neurologic condition themselves and appreciate help not only with identification of the neurologic disorder but also in management. In the current ICU environment—rapidly changing and becoming more complicated each year—it is appropriate to ask who might be best suited to assess these patients. If we are going to fully appreciate the complexity of consulting in the ICU, there is much to be said for a specialty that concentrates on providing a comprehensive neurology consult in the ICU. Expertise is warranted in the assessment of neuroimaging. In some patients, electroencephalography (EEG) monitoring and treatment of unexpected nonconvulsive status epilepticus are required and necessitate special expertise.[6,8] One can successfully argue for the presence of a core group of neurohospitalists or neurointensivists providing such services. Neurocritical care, as a distinct specialty, provides the expertise of consultation in other ICUs, and close communication with intensivists must be beneficial to the patient.

These ICU consults are often urgent consults. Some may think that one can simply pick up the phone and ask the expert (or whoever might be considered an expert). In many intensive care practices, it seems often easier to call a consultant than to ask for a formal consult. Both parties often agree that some type of advice will pragmatically direct testing or treatment. For the intensivist, there may be other immediately pressing priorities in the complex care of the patient, so a new neurologic problem is best solved quickly.

Any of the neurology "curbside consultations" in the ICU are indeed simple phone calls for a simple question, but some of these questions should probably generate a formal consult. These so-called curbsides are a set of questions that pertain to critical illness and often involve interpretation of a computed tomography (CT) scan of the brain, questions about EEG interpretation or need for EEG monitoring, how to manage neurologic medications such as antiepileptic drugs, how to assess the risk of anticoagulation, and how to interpret specific neurologic manifestations of acute neurologic disease. Consultants should generally avoid the practice of phone calls and curbsides, but if it occurs the neurologist will have to consider the following questions: How can I best ask pointed questions? Am I able to provide advice with limited information and without having the opportunity to examine the patient? Am I confident enough to dismiss or diagnose certain CT scan abnormalities? Does this clinical problem in all likelihood require a close follow-up and thus a formal consultation?

Acute (STAT) consults in the ICU are the most challenging consults in the hospital. First, decisions may have to be made in an evolving situation and the primary diagnosis may be unclear and puzzling. Second, neurologic examination can be compromised when patients are markedly swollen, jaundiced, immobile, or bruised or have major operation sites or an open chest. Moreover, the neuroimaging and electrophysiology findings may not be particularly helpful.

Once a full consult is established, any neurologist may consider the following: Are the neurologic findings commensurating with the cause and degree of critical illness? Are the focal findings real or difficult to judge? How is neuroimaging or electrophysiology best interpreted in the setting of critical illness? Are there urgent treatment options or treatment adjustments that may not have been considered? Does this neurologic manifestation set the patient back permanently? Can I reliably provide an opinion on the likelihood of the functional status of the patient in the near future, and what prognostic certainty could put an end to the full-court press, constantly escalating care?

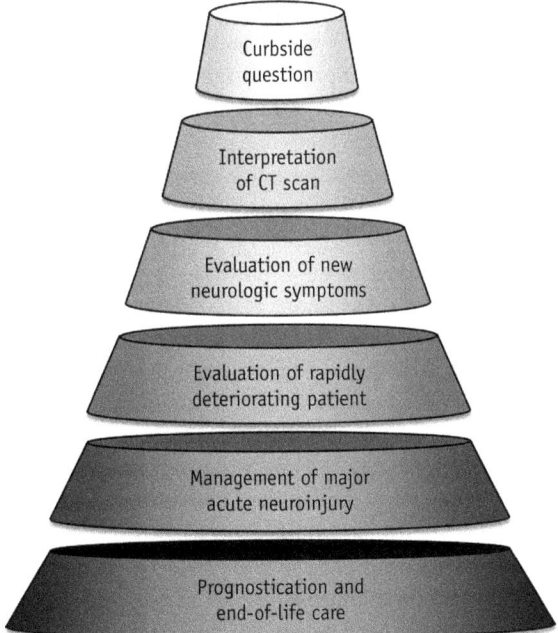

Figure 1.1 The complexity of a neurology consult in the ICU.

This introductory chapter presents the general principles and practice of consultative neurology in medical and surgical ICUs.

Consultation may evolve from being asked a simple question to being physically present to continuously manage an acute injury to the brain or the spine, and it may even involve palliation and end-of-life discussions. There is a spectrum of close participation with the consulting neurologist (Figure 1.1).

Principles

One of the first core principle is to determine whether the problem can be handled as a curbside or requires a formal consultation. The immediate concern, before assessment of the medical record, is the reliability of the initial piece of information provided by a colleague physician. Unsurprisingly, audits in some studied interactions have shown that the accuracy of the information provided can be quite poor.[4] (A neurosurgical referral in the United Kingdom found common inaccuracies and poor follow-up after advise was given.[5]) This inadequacy can be explained not only by differences in expertise (the so-called "wrongly billed" patient) but also by changing patient parameters.

The term *curbside* is understood here as a physician–neurologist interaction undertaken to obtain advice that would not require a full consult with a comprehensive patient evaluation and examination. It may consist of a phone call (most often), an e-mail, or a hallway conversation (less often). These interactions do involve expert advice ("May I run a case by you?") and may involve interpretation of neuroimaging results ("Can you look at this scan?"). Naturally, these curbsides may lead to a formal consultation when the situation seems "confusing or baffling" to the consultant.

The neurologist has to determine whether the question asked (Table 1.1) is too complicated to answer over the phone, but in the new digital world easy access to electronic medical records has significantly improved these conversations. Notes can now be reviewed quickly, tests can be retrieved, and laboratory results can be compared over time or even put in graph form. Infusates are readily available. Even the patient's vital signs, mode of mechanical ventilation, and intravenous (IV) medications are accessible without difficulty from any portal or wireless device. Neurologic examination may almost seem like an afterthought and may sometimes be considered unnecessary by the requesting physician.

A typical reason for a curbside is to determine the need for a formal consult. When all subspecialties are considered, formal neurologic consultations are more often pursued than curbside consultations.[13] (It is the same with curbsides involving infectious disease consultants: A simple inquiry about the best use of antibiotics or the best combination of antibiotics is often the main question, but most consultants want more involvement in the case presented.[17]) Curbsides are different from telemedicine consultations, because they are more focused on a single question and provide no remuneration. There are also legal risks, which may be truncated if such a conversation is adequately documented and if there is a conversion of the curbside into a consult.[7] However, curbsides may prove to be congenial to the problem of lacking neurologic expertise in hospitals with ICUs.[14,15,24]

The second core principle is to see the patient immediately (rather than the next day). There are several reasons to avoid an initial non-reaction and belated visit. First, the neurologic illness may have gone unrecognized and may require immediate intervention (e.g., increasing intracranial pressure, meningoencephalitis, undiagnosed myasthenic crisis). Second, the entire clinical picture may be unclear, and neurologic expertise may point toward the right diagnosis (e.g., sepsis due to epidural spinal abscess). Third, and more delicately, treatments may be inappropriate, incomplete, or incorrect. Neurologic illness in a critically ill patient remains difficult to recognize. I have seen a good amount of failure to recognize reversible causes of coma, failure to recognize spinal cord injury, and failure to recognize aphasia and failure to recognize fluctuating stupor or agitation from seizures. I have been blindsided too and misjudgments happen easily, even in the best-equipped and staffed ICUs.

Table 1.1 **Reasons for a Consult in the Intensive Care Unit**

- Acutely comatose
- Failure to awaken after resuscitation
- Acute focal deficit
- Acute agitation (with escalating drug use)
- Acute movements
- Generalized muscle weakness
- Unexplained neuroimaging findings
- Unexplained electroencephalography findings

The third core principle is to get up to par regarding the current pharmacologic management of critically ill patients. This part is demanding. Neurologists should appreciate the pharmacology of sedative drugs and the use of analgesic drugs in order to provide a better assessment.[3,23] Reconstruction of the pharmacodynamics and pharmacokinetics might be useful but is complicated because of multiorgan failure. Simple calculation of the metabolic half-life and the time to clearance may not be sufficient in determining a confounding effect on level of consciousness. This particularly applies to severely jaundiced patients who have recently been administered a good dose of benzodiazepine or a narcotic drug such as fentanyl. Frequently, there is an underestimation of the prolonged washout of these drugs and patients may look much worse because of it.[16]

Treatment of critical illness and its complications requires a vast array of drugs, and drug clearance may also be prolonged due to drug interaction (Table 1.2). Known interactions include midazolam with barbiturates and opioids with benzodiazepines. It is also well known that clearance of benzodiazepines is much delayed with prolonged IV infusions causing these drugs and metabolites to accumulate. Sedation and analgesia are commonly considered in restless patients who are likely experiencing pain after surgery. The liberal use of fentanyl infusions in surgical patients is often impressive—to put it mildly. Neurologists are taken aback (if they recognize it) by the phenomenal doses used (and continued) in cases of cardiac or complex orthopedic surgery. Most doses are much higher than in standard infusions (e.g., fentanyl infusion 1.5 mg/kg/min). Of course, these doses have major benefits, reducing pain-related myocardial demand ischemia and greatly facilitating postoperative mechanical

Table 1.2 **Drugs that Confound Neurologic Examination in Critical Illness**

Drug	Ideal half-life (hours)	Known interactions or organ failure prolonging elimination
Fentanyl*	2–5	Clonidine Metoclopramide Cimetidine Liver failure
Midazolam	4	Diltiazem Fungicides
Lorazepam	10–20	Opioids Liver failure
Propofol	0.5	No known interactions
Dexmedetomidine	0.5–1	No prolongation with organ failure
Vecuronium**	0.25	Corticosteroids Metronidazole

*Other opioids have comparable half-lives.
**Rocuronium (used for intubation) has rapid elimination (30 minutes).

ventilation. It is therefore often not a simple measure to advise to simply withhold the medication in order to have an unconfounded neurologic examination.

Muscle relaxants are either nondepolarizing (pancuronium, vecuronium, and atracurium) or depolarizing (succinylcholine)—this distinction refers to what occurs at the motor end-plate receptor units. Administration of a depolarizing drug opens the sodium–potassium (Na/K) channels, and no antidote can be effective, precisely because the channels are open. Nondepolarizing drugs compete with acetylcholine, and a drug such as neostigmine can reduce breakdown of acetylcholine (and thus increase the effect of acetylcholine through competition). The effect of succinylcholine can be prolonged, mostly because of a large administered dose (or a very uncommon genetic defect that prevents breakdown of succinylcholine). Use of muscle relaxants has decreased substantially now that ICU physicians appreciate that its use may be related to ICU-acquired weakness (Chapter 7). In any event, when in doubt, consulting neurologists can ask for (or perform) a train-of-four stimulation with a bedside peripheral nerve stimulator to record whether blockade is still present (i.e., fewer than four twitches).

The fourth core principle is to recognize that assessment is definitely confounded in patients who have recently undergone therapeutic hypothermia. Neurologic examination maybe impossible to perform initially in this circumstance, but it also may be problematic later. Therapeutic hypothermia is mostly used in the treatment of patients who have remained comatose after CPR, and it requires a combination of sedatives and neuromuscular blockers to mute shivering or any other sense of discomfort. These drugs are eliminated in a delayed fashion even after the patient has obtained a normal temperature. The kidney and liver that eliminate these drugs may have been seriously injured during prolonged resuscitation.

The fifth core principle is to recognize the patient's cause of illness and severity of illness. Any neurologist—as a result of frequent consultation—can develop this expertise. Having ICU knowledge will help one avoid getting lost in a maze of tremendous medical complexity and allow one to sort out the most important features. Direct communication with the attending physicians can decrease evaluation time and might reveal important intraoperative complications such as hypotension or even CPR. Medical ICUs usually admit patients with acute hypoxic hypercarbic respiratory failure (often with preexisting chronic obstructive pulmonary disease), sepsis, and intoxications. Often, new complications on top of the primary illness result in long stays in the ICU with added management of infection, acid-base disorders, and electrolyte abnormalities. Therefore, a consult involves a multifaceted situation that requires one to carefully parse out the main problems.

Consults in surgical and trauma ICUs are often related to diagnostic evaluation of new spinal cord injury and traumatic brain injury, but in most instances, other specialties have been involved (i.e., neurosurgery). Consults in coronary care units have evolved into co-management because many patients after CPR, and often after emergency coronary catheterization for acute coronary disease, are subjected to therapeutic hypothermia; in such cases, neurologists are closely involved with assessment of the degree of anoxic-ischemic injury. Coronary care units may ask that the neurohospitalist or neurointensivist direct the majority of neurologic care. A special category is consultation in the transplant recipient, which may have already started before transplantation. These situations are very complex, and a separate chapter is available in another volume of this series (*Handling Difficult Situations*). In this volume, we more closely look at the management of brain edema after fulminant hepatic failure. Decisions (e.g., ICP monitoring) are very difficult here.

Finally, the sixth core principle is to decisively prognosticate when possible, but to hold back when information conflicts. It is a common misperception that persistent coma in critical illness (i.e., coma lasting days) warrants swift withdrawal (or de-escalation) of critical care, particularly when families seek out the neurologist and cannot see a benefit from all the interventions. Consulting neurologists may be directly asked by family members about the rationale for care provided and may be placed in a compromising position. Participation in family discussions by the consulting neurologist with the entire team should be the norm, even if it is disruptive to other responsibilities such as daily rounds. Resolution of conflicts or arbitration may be needed, but most conferences are cordial, clarifying and clear to all family members. The role of neurologists here cannot be overemphasized, and their presence is often appreciated by the attending intensivist or surgeon.

In Practice

Whether faced with a curbside question ("Do you have a second?") or confronted with an urgent consult, the neurologist often sees the degree of difficulty ratcheting up within hours. The ICU consult is a matter of finding the right pieces of information quickly. How does this work in practice, and how should neurologists proceed?

CURBSIDES IN THE INTENSIVE CARE UNIT

What are the commonly asked questions that are often dealt with over the phone? Curbsides can be problematic if the question seems to merely scratch the surface. The decision to not convert a curbside into a consult should not be taken lightly—particularly for patients who just have been admitted to the ICU. Often, more than a simple yes or no answer is needed (Figure 1.2). In this section, the 10 most commonly asked questions are discussed.

Can You Look at This CT Scan?
Usually, the value of CT scans in critically ill patients is marginal and there are few surprising findings. Increased use of neuroimaging will lead to increased recognition of nonspecific signs that may lead to increased consultation. Many of these consultations can be deferred after review of the cases. However, CT scans may reveal clinically relevant lesions. Most (neuro)radiologists alert the attending physician personally, but others just dictate a note, leaving the critical care physician to recognize the urgency. Often, the finding is an unexpected lesion that could be serious and indicative of a more systemic process (e.g., infectious

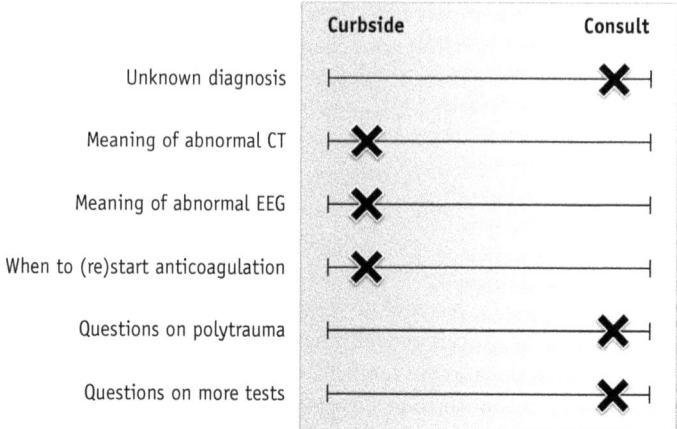

Figure 1.2 Curbside or consult?

emboli to the brain in a patient with infectious endocarditis). The challenge here is to decide whether a more formal consult is needed, one that may even include a neurosurgeon if surgery might be required. The need for an acute neurosurgery consult is underappreciated by many (for a chapter specifically focused on acute neurosurgical consultations, see another volume in this series, *Handling Difficult Situations*).

The most important abnormalities to recognize as immediately urgent are the following: any new large lesion or new brain edema, any traumatic brain contusion particularly when the CT scan is a day old and the contusion may have expanded), any extracerebral hematoma, any hydrocephalus, and any mass lesion in the posterior fossa. An urgent magnetic resonance imaging (MRI) study may be needed to better define the abnormality and its impact on surrounding structures. And then there are the "zebras" or surprises. For example, I have seen instances of pituitary apoplexy after a major surgical procedure, and this small lesion can rapidly cause havoc and visual loss if not acted on quickly.

A CT scan may show an abnormality of uncertain significance. Hypodensities are frequently found in the cerebellum and in most instances, they represent an older infarct. Small lacunar infarcts in both cerebral hemispheres are common in patients with a metabolic syndrome and a medical complication that brought them to the ICU. Often, in polytrauma patients, the mere presence of small amounts of hemorrhage into parietooccipital sulci or some blood layering on the tentorium prompts a quick consultation. CT scans are often ordered for patients with acute change in responsiveness, new-onset delirium, or presumed focal signs, but then we can expect that incidental findings are common.

Can You Interpret This EEG?

The circumstances that surround critical illness could make the patient more vulnerable to seizures if there is an epileptogenic structural lesion. Yet, few patients in the ICU have seizures; many more have EEGs ordered. The clinical recognition of seizures is not easy, and seizures in the ICU may be observed by staff members who have difficulty recognizing different types of twitching movements. There is a tendency to mistake movements such as extensor posturing, dystonia, and shivering for a seizure. Syncope due to cardiac arrhythmia and a sudden blood pressure drop can cause backward eye-rolling, myoclonic twitches, tonic posturing, and slurring of speech. During a syncope, a brief period of staring may occur that is impossible to differentiate clinically from postictal confusion. Furthermore, myoclonic jerks are probably more common than seizures, simply because myokymias and myoclonus are well-known side effects of drugs frequently used in the ICU. Alcohol withdrawal seizures often occur in patients with a history of heavy drinking, who inevitably experience sobriety after ICU admission.

In most hospitals, an intensivist can order an EEG if there is a need to exclude seizures or to explain failure to awaken. Taken at random and with questionable indication, the yield of abnormal EEGs is very low and only results in overconsultation. In many instances, the EEG shows a nonspecific slowing or a medication effect. Triphasic waves or frontal intermittent rhythmic delta activity is often seen in patients with multiorgan failure; both are nonspecific (and definitively non-epileptogenic) findings. The most common misinterpretation of triphasic waves is non-convulsive status epilepticus (NCSE). With a rhythmic frequency greater than 1 per second, this pattern may be construed as NCSE only if there is additional evidence of extra spikes and less generalized background slowing. Absent reactivity of triphasic waves correlates with poor outcome.[22]

Do We Need Prolonged EEG Monitoring?

For patients in whom the EEG shows epileptiform activity, further monitoring may be necessary. Comatose patients treated for sepsis who are monitored and studied may be found to have electrographic seizures (present in 10%), periodic epileptic discharges (17%), or both.[20] NCSE can be confirmed with an EEG recording that demonstrates diffuse spike or polyspike and wave complexes at frequencies of 1–3 Hz. Many of these abnormalities are associated with a new neurologic injury. Furthermore, if NCSE is found, its management may not necessarily lead to better outcome.[21,25] In other words, indiscriminate use of continuous EEG monitoring in a medically or surgically critically ill patient is highly questionable and expensive, and if found after a major acute brain injury may not change outcome.

Does the Patient Have a Neurologic Cause for Failure to Wean from the Ventilator?

An almost universal question is whether failure of weaning is caused by a previously unappreciated and undiagnosed neurologic disorder. Electrodiagnostic tests such as electromyography may have been ordered but were nondiagnostic. This is a common curbside question and cannot be resolved with just a phone call. In most instances of failure to wean, these tests are not useful; the same applies to phrenic nerve testing and needle examination of the diaphragm. Many patients who are chronically ventilator dependent will have developed diaphragmatic atrophy—a phenomenon that starts rather quickly. Paradoxical and asynchronous breathing is observed when these patients with poor diaphragmatic endurance are briefly taken off the ventilator.

Most of the time, contraction of the diaphragm can be documented (with the use of bag-assisted deep inspiration) on ultrasound of the chest. Needle examination will document fibrillation potentials as a sign of muscular injury but often cannot definitively differentiate between a neurogenic and a muscular origin.

Bedside pulmonary function tests can be useful, but they require a major effort by the patient and may not be reliable. Patients with diaphragmatic weakness show a decrease in vital capacity when supine, but must be greater 25% from baseline to be called abnormal. Conversely, a normal supine vital capacity makes an inspiratory muscle weakness highly unlikely. A high maximal inspiratory pressure (>80 cm H_2O) makes neuromuscular respiratory failure unlikely, particularly in combination with a normal vital capacity. In many patients with a neurologic cause of respiratory weakness, there is associated generalized weakness.

The diagnosis of critical illness polyneuropathy requires confirmation with a nerve conduction study and needle examination. Again, needle examination of the diaphragm in a patient after a long period of mechanical ventilation and considerable atrophy may be difficult to interpret, and whether paradoxical breathing exists due to critical illness polyneuropathy is questionable.[18] In some patients, amyotrophic lateral sclerosis (ALS) is evident, such as when the patient presents with acute respiratory failure in end-stage ALS, and that by itself is worth a neurologist visit. Neurologists may provide an accurate explanation and help with future care and support.

How Do I "Clear" the Cervical Spine?

In any patient with polytrauma or a fall from a standing height, a collar may have been placed. Clearing of the cervical spine (i.e., confirming exclusion of cervical spine injury) requires examination in an alert patient to determine whether movement of the spine is painful. If this is not possible, an MRI of the spine is needed. But a recent study suggest that CT scan might be sufficient in an "obtunded" patient.[1] Evaluation of the spine should proceed with flexion and extension photographs (which should be proven normal) and with a multiplanar CT scan of the cervical spine. In any patient, a CT scan of the spine is necessary to exclude major injuries such as an odontoid fracture or other unstable fractures that could lead to an immediate neurologic deficit if the patient is not protected by a cervical collar. A full neurologic examination should involve flexion and extension, lateral rotation, and lateral flexion, and no pain should be elicited when the physician gently steers these movements by holding the patient's head with two hands —neurologists often ask neurosurgeons to do the examination and interpretation.

How Do I Manage Autonomic Storming?

Many patients with polytrauma and traumatic brain injury will develop a paroxysmal sympathetic hyperactivity syndrome (also known as autonomic storming), which leads to tachycardia, tachypnea, profuse sweating, and hypertensive spikes.[11] The treatment of choice is high-dose gabapentin (up to 2,400 mg daily), with intermittent doses of morphine, if necessary. The autonomic storming is often not recognized, and many patients will have had a battery of diagnostic tests that were all negative. This is one example of a condition that could be treated if recognized by a consulting neurologist.

How Do I Manage Fluctuating Blood Pressure in Spinal Cord Injury?
Fluctuating blood pressure in spinal cord injury is potentially problematic and can lead to marked shifts and instability. There is a consensus that mean arterial pressure values should be consistently greater than 65 mm Hg. Both extremes of blood pressure may occur, in which case patients may be treated by alternating use of fluid boluses and vasopressors or nicardipine infusions to overcome these autonomic fluctuations.

How Long Should I Continue Antiepileptic Drugs?
Antiepileptic drugs are provided prophylactically to many patients, particularly those in whom seizures have been observed. Because most newer antiepileptic drugs (i.e levetiracetam) are cleared during hemodialysis, a single dose should be administered after hemodialysis to patients who have a history of witnessed seizures. Prophylactic use of antiepileptic drugs in patients with an acute brain injury is a contentious issue. Administration for longer than 1 week is usually not warranted. Seizures in critically ill patients are often a single event, in which case long-term use of antiepileptic drugs is not warranted. Early seizures after traumatic brain injury may be best treated with levetiracetam for 4 weeks.

When Can I Start Anticoagulation?
Prophylactic subcutaneous heparin can be started 2 days after CT documentation of a stable cerebral hematoma or contusion. Although longterm anticoagulation can be restarted after an intracranial hemorrhage or contusion, the timing is unclear. Most experts would resume anticoagulation after an arbitrary 4 weeks, but this is ill advised in patients who are at high risk for embolization from a prosthetic valve, in whom oral anticoagulation has to be resumed after 7–10 days. Repeated echocardiograms (twice weekly) may allow better assessment of the potential risk because they may show valve dysfunction and strand formation, which may lead to initiation of IV heparin. In patients with deep venous thrombosis (with or without pulmonary emboli) after a recent cerebral hemorrhage or major hemorrhagic infarct we place an IVC filter and delay anticoagulation for 4 weeks (the risk of recurrent major pulmonary emboli pushing through an IVC filter is very low in the first 3–6 months; the risk of recurrent major hemorrhage in the brain possibly requiring surgery with full early anticoagulation is likely much higher).

Factors that increase the risk of recurrent intracranial hemorrhage are advanced age, poorly controlled hypertension, and prior hemorrhages. Any patient with atrial fibrillation, a metallic mitral valve, a high CHADS2 score for stroke risk, a left ventricular assist device, and an intracardiac thrombus documented by transesophageal echocardiography requires long term anticoagulation. In one recent study with mostly patients with atrial fibrillation and high CHADS2 score, median resumption after 30 days was not associated with more frequent rehemorrhage at a one-year follow-up mark.[12]

How Do I Provide Medication in Parkinson's Disease?
All patients with Parkinson's disease who have major abdominal surgery, whether elective or emergent, need to restart their Parkinson's disease medication. The problem here is that sudden withdrawal of Parkinson's drugs can lead to marked rigidity and

dysautonomia that can potentially jeopardize the patient's well-being. Adjustment of medication is seldom needed, and medication should be administered through a nasogastric tube as soon as the bowels function.

FORMAL CONSULTATIONS IN THE INTENSIVE CARE UNIT

Neurologic consultation for patients in medical and surgical ICUs is often prompted by altered consciousness, seizures, or the recent discovery of focal deficits. Neurologic evaluation often involves evaluation of a CT or MRI scan and, in approximately one third of the patients, interpretation of a routinely ordered EEG. In our preliminary study, benefits of ICU consults are substantial (Figure 1.3).[19] Diagnostic benefit was documented in a large proportion of patients, prognostic benefit in about one third, and treatment benefit in about one third.

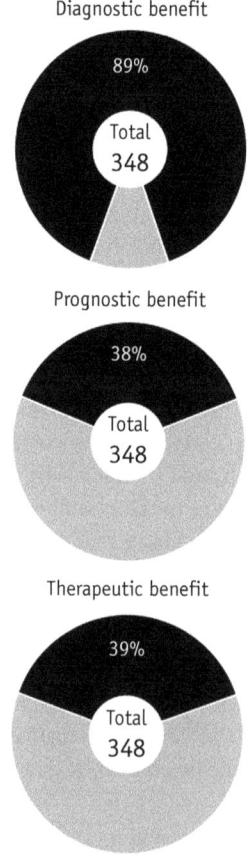

Figure 1.3 Summary of review of ICU consultations at Mayo Clinic Campus Hospitals. (Adapted from Mittal et al., 2014.[19])

In our experience, a mixed encephalopathy is found in about one third of patients, followed by stroke, seizures, anoxic-ischemic injury, central nervous system infection, spinal cord pathology, and a variety of other disorders. We have found a high incidence of posterior reversible encephalopathy syndrome (PRES) and a growing incidence of serotonin syndrome and cefepime encephalopathy. Neuromuscular weakness was assessed in approximately 1 of every 10 patients. In most cases, the patients had been admitted with acute respiratory failure, marked weight loss, and weakness. A critical illness myopathy was usually found. An undiagnosed neurologic disorder was found in only a handful of patients.

The major reasons for consultation in this study included the assessment of new-onset seizures, generalized weakness, delirium and other states of altered awareness and coma, postresuscitation encephalopathy, and, infrequently, a neurologic complication after vascular surgery that involved the spinal cord. Neurologic complications after organ transplantation have declined over the last decade and are now incidental consultations.

Before discussing the major critical consults in this monograph, it may be useful to summarize a general approach of assessment. First, one should at least obtain some sense of the circumstance in which the patient was found (apneic, cyanotic, or actively seizing with forced eye deviation), whether there was a prior illness or any known constitutional symptoms, and whether there were any recent medication adjustments or newly started drugs, particularly antibiotics such as cefepime.

Next, one should evaluate whether focal findings are present. Acute hemiparesis in a critically ill patient is most commonly caused by an acute ischemic or hemorrhagic stroke or a developing contusion in a patient with traumatic head injury. An acute hemiparesis is usually flaccid throughout, but in others muscle testing is required to find a pyramidal pattern belonging to an upper motor neuron lesion. However, a lesion from motor cortex to pons will result in a hemiparesis with the arm more involved than the leg, a pattern that is not seen in upper cervical spinal cord lesions, and reflexes become brisk soon after onset. Acute paraparesis or tetraparesis indicates a spinal cord lesion and may be caused by a compressive lesion (e.g., epidural abscess or hematoma) or an intraspinal lesion (e.g., spinal cord infarction or contusion). A sensory level is usually sought; if a level is identified, an attempt is made to further localize the lesion to a particular segment of the spinal cord. Acute monoplegia could point toward a brachial or lumbosacral plexus lesion, particularly in a patient with polytrauma. It can be caused by direct trauma, operative stretch during chest surgery, or compression (e.g., psoas hematoma). If hemiparesis involves one extremity, it can be almost impossible to distinguish between upper motor neuron and lower motor neuron involvement.

Most movement disorders in critical illness are myoclonus or tremors. Dystonia or chorea is rarely seen. An unusual finding remains dystonia that is classically associated with metoclopramide or ondansetron use or the use of selective serotonin reuptake inhibitors (SSRIs). Myoclonus in a comatose patient is most often associated with an anoxic-ischemic injury that has

Table 1.3 **Essentials of Neurology Consultation in the Intensive Care Unit**

- Assess details on severity of critical illness
- Assess blood pressure and extent of blood pressure support
- Assess drug administration over 5–7 days
- Verify onset of symptoms with nursing staff
- Assess major confounders (therapeutic hypothermia, acute metabolic derangements, and acid-base abnormalities)
- Assess for possible movements, twitching, new rigidity
- Assess for drugs strongly related to delirium, movement disorders

resulted in diffuse laminal necrosis. In any other patient, myoclonus is often seen in the setting of new antimicrobial use, in particular cefepime or an SSRI. Myoclonus is a common occurrence after a large dose of opioids or calcium channel blockers. Tremors are common in any patient with multiorgan failure and are not clinically relevant.

Table 1.3 describes how to proceed with an acute neurology consult in the ICU. A consult is concluded with adequate documentation of neurologic findings, impression, and explanation. A preliminary diagnosis is made, and tests are suggested. The attending team should be asked to call when the results are available or some sort of follow-through is needed to obtain results quickly. Recommendations may vary from a single advice to more detailed treatments in the unit until the problem is resolved (e.g., control of intracranial pressure, seizure control). End-of-life care by the neurologist is expected and common. Details on how to proceed with family conversations are found in a separate volume of this series (*Communicating Prognosis*).

Putting It All Together

- Neurologic consultation in the ICU requires a broad base of medical knowledge.
- Neurologic consultation provides diagnostic, therapeutic, and prognostic advice.
- Neurologic consultation in the ICU may change the approach to the patient.
- Neurologic consultation often involves assessment of unresponsiveness or seizures.
- Neurologic consultation may detect an unsuspected neurologic disorder.
- Neurologic consultation involves end-of-life decisions for some patients.

By the Way

- CT scans in confused delirious patients often show incidental findings.
- The incidence of PRES is rising in ICUs.
- EEGs are usually more confusing than valuable in a drowsy patient.
- Early diffuse weakness in ICU is often undiagnosed ALS.
- Late diffuse weakness in ICU is often critical illness polyneuromyopathy.

> **Consulting in the Neuro ICU by the Numbers**
>
> - ~50% of ICU consults are for altered consciousness.
> - ~25% of ICU consults are for coma after CPR.
> - ~15% of ICU consults are for movements, twitching, or seizures.
> - ~10% of ICU consults are for generalized muscle weakness.
> - ~5% of ICU consults are for "new" CT scan abnormality.

References

1. Badhiwala JH, Lai CK, Alhazzani W, et al. Cervical spine clearance in obtunded patients after blunt traumatic injury: a systematic review. *Ann Intern Med* 2015;162: 429–437.
2. Bleck TP, Smith MC, Pierre-Louis SJ, et al. Neurologic complications of critical medical illnesses. *Crit Care Med* 1993;21:98–103.
3. Brust JCM. *Neurotoxic Side Effects of Prescription Drugs*. 2nd ed. Boston: Butterworth-Heinemann, 1996.
4. Burden M, Sarcone E, Keniston A, et al. Prospective comparison of curbside versus formal consultations. *J Hosp Med* 2013;8:31–35.
5. Cartmill M, White BD. Telephone advice for neurosurgical referrals: who assumes duty of care? *Br J Neurosurg* 2001;15:453–455.
6. Claassen J, Taccone FS, Horn P, et al. Recommendations on the use of EEG monitoring in critically ill patients: consensus statement from the neurointensive care section of the ESICM. *Intensive Care Med* 2013;39:1337–1351.
7. Cotton VR. Legal risks of "curbside" consults. *Am J Cardiol* 2010;106:135–138.
8. Firosh Khan S, Ashalatha R, Thomas SV, Sarma PS. Emergent EEG is helpful in neurology critical care practice. *Clin Neurophysiol* 2005;116:2454–2459.
9. Howard RS. Neurological problems on the ICU. *Clin Med* 2007;7:148–153.
10. Hughes CG, Patel MB, Pandharipande PP. Pathophysiology of acute brain dysfunction: what's the cause of all this confusion? *Curr Opin Crit Care* 2012;18:518–526.
11. Hughes JD, Rabinstein AA. Early diagnosis of paroxysmal sympathetic hyperactivity in the ICU. *Neurocrit Care* 2014;20:454–459.
12. Kuramatsu B, Gerner ST, Schellinger PD, et al. Anticoagulant reversal, blood pressure levels, and anticoagulant levels and resumption in patients with anticoagulation-related intracerebral hemorrhage. *JAMA* 2015;313:824–836.
13. Kuo D, Gifford DR, Stein MD. Curbside consultation practices and attitudes among primary care physicians and medical subspecialists. *JAMA* 1998;280:905–909.
14. Lilly CM, McLaughlin JM, Zhao H, et al. A multicenter study of ICU telemedicine reengineering of adult critical care. *Chest* 2014;145:500–507.
15. Lilly CM, Zubrow MT, Kempner KM, et al. Critical care telemedicine: evolution and state of the art. *Crit Care Med* 2014;42:2429–2436.
16. Makii JM, Mirski MA, Lewin JJ 3rd. Sedation and analgesia in critically ill neurologic patients. *J Pharm Pract* 2010;23:455–469.
17. Manian FA, McKinsey DS. A prospective study of 2,092 "curbside" questions asked of two infectious disease consultants in private practice in the midwest. *Clin Infect Dis* 1996;22:303–307.
18. Maramattom BV, Wijdicks EF. Acute neuromuscular weakness in the intensive care unit. *Crit Care Med* 2006;34:2835–2841.

19. Mittal MK, Kashyap R, Herasevich V, Rabinstein A, Wijdicks EFM. Do patients in a medical or surgical ICU benefit from a neurologic consultation? *Int J Neurosci* 2014 Sep 10 [Epub ahead of print].
20. Oddo M, Carrera E, Claassen J, Mayer SA, Hirsch LJ. Continuous electroencephalography in the medical intensive care unit. *Crit Care Med* 2009;37:2051–2056.
21. Rabinstein AA. Continuous electroencephalography in the medical ICU. *Neurocrit Care* 2009;11:445–446.
22. Sutter R, Stevens RD, Kaplan PW. Significance of triphasic waves in patients with acute encephalopathy: a nine-year cohort study. *Clin Neurophysiol* 2013;124:1952–1958.
23. Wijdicks EFM. *Neurologic Complications of Critical Illness*. 3rd ed. New York: Oxford University Press, 2009.
24. Wilcox ME, Adhikari NK. The effect of telemedicine in critically ill patients: systematic review and meta-analysis. *Crit Care* 2012;16:R127.
25. Young GB. Continuous EEG monitoring in the ICU: challenges and opportunities. *Can J Neurol Sci* 2009;36 Suppl 2:S89–91.

2

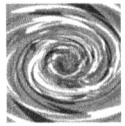

Acute Confusion in the Critically Ill

Critically ill patients—by the nature of their condition—lose their perceptual abilities. Some patients become wild, thrash around, move their head from side to side, pick, buck, yell to an imaginary person, and generally appear very uncomfortable or perhaps even terrified. Breathing may be increasingly labored, and blood pressure and heart rate rise significantly. A delirious patient is literally "off the track." Because minor presentations of confusion are ubiquitously present in intensive care units (ICUs), some threshold must be crossed to trigger calling in a neurologist or psychiatrist. There is no question that acute confusion, or "altered mental state" (a very indistinct and altogether avoidable term), is not only the most common but also overused reason for a neurologic consultation.[2,4]

Critically ill patients are routinely monitored for the development of delirium, and nursing rating scales are in place. This is particularly useful with patients who have a history of alcohol or drug use, but such a history may be held back or forcefully denied.[19] Neurologists and, more recently, neurointensivists see many patients with new-onset confusion. Some have obvious new neurologic findings, such as a hemiparesis or a speech impediment. In a large proportion of patients, neither electroencephalography (EEG) nor neuroimaging contributes to determining the cause of an acute confusional state, but both add considerably to the cost of care. Causes are rarely found, and many patients improve after a short pharmaceutical intervention. However, an acutely confused critically ill patient may harbor an acute neurologic disorder that can be immediately problematic.

This chapter addresses the following questions: How do we define and monitor an acute confusional state or delirium? How can we best make sense of a confused and fidgety patient? How can we best bring some clarity in the terminology? What initial considerations and laboratory tests are necessary? How can we best manage agitated patients, and for how long?

Data suggest that there are long-term consequences of unchecked delirium in a critically ill patient.[5,24,26] An unexplained observation is that delirium is associated with increased mortality but none of the studies in which delirium was aggressively treated have shown an improved mortality rate. Most physicians believe that treatment with potent sedative drugs should be swift, because there are few other options to calm the patient.

Principles

Delirium can be better conceptualized, better monitored, and better treated in the ICU. Structured tests are helpful, but delirium or any type of new acute confusion is usually defined by its principal symptoms: restlessness, disorientation, lack of sustained attention, and frightful screams. Is it easy to recognize? Yes it should be.

MECHANISMS OF DELIRIUM

Delirium is such a complex disorder that it is not a surprising that we know little to nothing. Risk factors are present in some ICUs and not in others.[12,37] Generally, the effect of critical illness on neuronal circuitry is not understood—all that has been proposed seems either too far-fetched or purely speculative. Part of the problem is that studies involve heterogenic patients, so that many of the observations may apply, for example, only to patients who have a sepsis syndrome. All of the pathologic or pathophysiologic pathways in delirium are unknown or assumed to be a result of neurotransmitter changes. Anticholinergic drugs do increase the risk of delirium, so it is probable that acetylcholine pathways are involved. Similar observations have been found with use of dopaminergic drugs or γ-aminobutyric acid–ergic (GABAergic) drugs that enhance alertness but, in high doses, can also cause delirium. Excess norepinephrine activity or an increased noradrenergic state may easily impair attention and cause anxiety and the hyperactivity seen in delirium. Other pathways in the genesis of delirium may involve stress hormones, because high-dose corticosteroids can produce "steroid psychosis."

Further evidence that neurotransmitters are involved is that certain drugs improve agitation, either through stimulation or by "toning down" these neurotransmittors.[34] Examples are quetiapine and olanzapine with serotonin, dexmedetomidine with noradrenaline, propofol with gamma-aminobutyric acid (GABA) and ketamine with N-methyl-d-aspartate (NMDA). Haloperidol is an effective antidopaminergic drug (Table 2.1).

An equally important core principle is that it is useful to understand how sedative agents cause their sedative effect. First, all opioids work through interactions

Table 2.1 **Drugs Linked to Neurotransmitter Pathways**

Neurotransmitter	Drug	Effect on agitation
Dopamine	Haloperidol	↓
Acetylcholine	Rivastigmine, donepezil	↑
Serotonin	Quetiapine, olanzapine	↓
Noradrenaline	Clonidine, dexmedetomidine	↓
N-methyl-D-aspartate (NMDA)	Ketamine	↓
Melatonin	Melatonin	↓

with the opioid receptors and their various subtypes. Because these opioid receptors are ubiquitous in the body, opioids can cause not only analgesia but also respiratory depression, gastrointestinal hypomotility, and hypotension. Drugs that are μ-opioid receptor agonists include fentanyl, morphine, and remifentanil. The benzodiazepines are GABA$_A$ receptor agonists. Lorazepam has a long-acting effect, as opposed to midazolam, which is short-acting. Upregulation of the GABA receptors may reduce alertness, because GABA activates a hypothalamic structure called the ventrolateral preoptic nucleus, causing patients to become sleepy. This structure is the main target of most of the sedative drugs, such as the benzodiazepines and propofol. It is therefore apparent that benzodiazepines could treat delirium well but why benzodiazepines in a dose-dependent relation cause later delirium remains poorly understood.[23] The barbiturates are also GABA$_A$ receptor agonists, including thiopental, pentobarbital, and phenobarbital. This may also apply to propofol, although the true mechanism is unresolved. All drugs that have an inhibitory effect on the neurotransmitter GABA cause anterograde amnesia. Finally, α_2-agonists such as clonidine and dexmedetomidine can also be used for sedation, anxiolysis, and analgesia.[14] Dexmedetomidine has a much higher affinity for the α_2-receptor than clonidine, but there is only a mild effect on the level of arousal.

Apart from a direct effect on neurotransmitters, the brain may be challenged by reduced cerebral blood flow, such as in septic shock. However, there is very little convincing evidence to support an ischemic pathway that could eventually lead to neuronal apoptosis. Inflammatory markers such as tumor necrosis factor and Toll-like receptor are activated in sepsis and can activate microglial cells, but again this pathway may be operative only in delirium associated with septic encephalopathy. Whether inflammatory markers such as interleukin 6, interleukin 8, C-reactive protein, and procalcitonin are related to delirium is neither fully established nor well studied.

Is there an anatomic substrate for agitated delirium? Patients with an ischemic stroke and concomitant delirium have provided some possible insight, but most understanding has been derived from lesions in the limbic cortex or frontal regions. Lesions in the caudate nucleus can cause severe agitation (but also periods of extreme quietness) because connecting fibers to the frontal lobes are interrupted. Left temporal lesions can cause a wild, talkative patient, but this may not be much different from typical Wernicke aphasia. The main challenge is to recognize one of the more defined agnosias manifesting as "disorientation." There may be an impairment of visual-spatial task (right posterior parietal cortex), anosognosia (unawareness for hemiparesis), or severe amnesia (parahippocampus).[1,35] Autopsy findings in patients who were delirious do not provide satisfactory answers, because critically ill patients are a heterogeneous population, and many other factors may play a role.[15] Moreover, abnormalities involving the frontal cortex, basal ganglia, and thalamus are widespread.[38]

CLASSIFICATION OF CONFUSION

It is immediately obvious that the terminology is confusing in itself.[27,33] How does a psychiatrist or neurologist define delirium, and how is this different from the definition put forth by an intensivist? Many patients with renal or hepatic encephalopathy show daytime sleeping and nighttime agitation, also known as *sundowning*. Typically, delirium has several disturbed components, including arousal, language, perception, orientation, mood, and sleep. Restlessness is associated with pallor, sweating, and tachycardia, but also with wide pupils. This occurs most often after withdrawal of stimulants or central nervous system depressants such as alcohol. Most patients are hyperaroused, language is incoherent and rambling, and there is little comprehensible speech output. Orientation to time is impaired first, and impairment of orientation to place comes later. The mood may include anger and aggression.

Neurologists have long labeled patients who are not responding normally as somnolent, encephalopathic, drowsy, disoriented, or, when agitated, delirious. Delirium often has been diagnosed when confusion is associated with autonomic symptoms such as profuse sweating, muscle twitching, and fidgety movements that may include more targeted movements such as pulling lines and catheters (Figure 2.1).

There has been a serious attempt to reduce the number of designations, and some have categorized delirium as hyperactive, hypoactive, or mixed. Others have not been satisfied with this terminology and have introduced *subsyndromal delirium*, a state that lies between no delirium and clinical delirium.[21] Simplification of the terminology has its benefits, but it reduces the recognition of clear neurologic symptomatology. It has been proposed to define *hypoactive delirium* as a state characterized by less attention and paucity of movement, as opposed to *hyperactive delirium*, which is characterized by increased attention, agility, and exaggerated response to simple stimuli.[8-10] *Mixed forms* are defined as a combination of hypoactive and hyperactive delirium. If these "definitions" are used, studies have found that hyperactive delirium is far less common than hypoactive delirium or a mixed form. Hypoactive delirium has also been called *quiet delirium*, but it remains one of the most problematic designations to accept for a neurologist. It is uncertain how much drowsiness or lack of responsiveness is needed to indicate a diagnosis of hypoactive delirium, and many neurologists ask, what patients in an ICU would *not* fulfill these simple criteria? Any drowsy patient lacks concentration and attention and is unable to think clearly.

Although the term *encephalopathy* may not be ideal, it is much better understood than "hypoactive delirium." Naming encephalopathic patients in a hypoactive or quiet delirium would dramatically increase the prevalence and perhaps could also increase unnecessary treatment. One can also easily imagine that a patient with hypoactive delirium might harbor a central nervous system infection, nonconvulsive status epilepticus, a new metabolic derangement such as hyperammonemia, or a major side effect of a recently administered drug. How about the patient in a quiet delirium who exhibits facial twitching, eye deviation, or, in less common situations, cortical blindness (a presentation in patients with posterior reversible encephalopathy syndrome)? And who wants to miss abulia in a patient with an acute frontal lobe infarct? Moreover, I suspect that most consulting neurologists would want to continue to use the term *encephalopathy* in association with dysfunction of specific organs (see Chapter 3) and use the term *agitated delirium*.

Acute Confusion in the Critically Ill 21

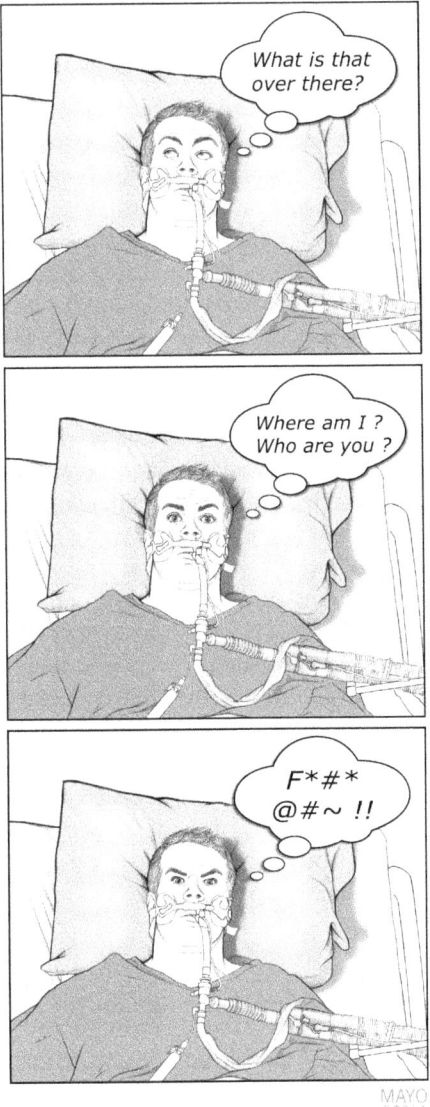

Figure 2.1 Illustration of agitated patients.

How can we best summarize examination findings? Several complex nursing scales have been developed, the most useful of which is the Confusion Assessment Method for the Intensive Care Unit (CAM-ICU).[17,28] This scale has been validated, but many of the tests do not consist of a detailed neurologic examination and largely focus on comprehension of language (Tables 2.2–2.4). One could argue that the neurologic examination in a confused patient should at least include testing recall, naming of three unrelated objects (e.g., "car," "Mr. Johnson," and "tunnel"), attention, repeating a series of digits (e.g., a telephone number), calculation (e.g., counting down from 100 by subtracting 7), and also writing and reading a complete sentence. If possible, copying a cube and following a more complex command (e.g., "Before you point to the ceiling, point toward your nose") should also be included.

Equally important is the question whether a full mental status examination can be used to further examine the patient who is in a confusional state. Most of the screening tests evaluate nothing more than attention and distractibility; they vary from counting backward from 20 to having the patient name months forward and backward or indicate the letter "A" in a random list of letters or a specific sentence.[7] Obviously, impaired attention will markedly influence the testing of other cognitive domains. Nonetheless, there is an obligation to test for clear neurologic abnormalities that may not have been examined with sufficient detail (Table 2.5).

For a patient with aphasia, fluency, naming, repetition, comprehension, and praxis should be tested. This may include recognition of paraphasic errors (phonemic or semantic); naming of an object (e.g., a wedding ring); repetition of a phrase (e.g., "It is a nice day today"); notice of comprehension, often with yes-and-no questions (e.g., "Am I wearing glasses?"); reading and writing; and praxis (e.g., "Show me your teeth. Buff your cheeks. Wave goodbye."). Patients who are apraxic have an inability to copy or pantomime. Abulia can be tested using grasp, snout reflex, or motor impersistence. When the patient is neglecting a visual field is important and can sometimes be determined only by more complex tests such as copying of geometric designs or clock drawing.

A simple test of executive function is the Oral Trail Making Test, in which the patient is asked to name letters of the alphabet and add a number for each (e.g., A1, B2, C3, D4, E5). Neglect in a patient who is agnostic is important and would have to be determined by finding neglect of the left side, cortical blindness, or prosopagnosia. Each of these abnormalities can identify damage to specific regions of the brain and may indicate an infarction, a hemorrhage abscess, or a metastasis that is less clearly identifiable on the computed tomography (CT) scan

Table 2.2 **Richmond Agitation Sedation Scale for the Assessment of Depth of Sedation**

+4	Very combative, violent, dangerous to staff
+3	Pulling catheters and tubes, aggressive
+2	Frequent nonpurposeful movements, fights ventilator
+1	Anxious, but movements not aggressive or vigorous
0	Alert and calm
−1	Awakes (eye contact) for >10 sec in response to voice
−2	Awakes (eye contact) for <10 sec in response to voice
−3	Eye opening or movements in response to voice without eye contact
−4	No response to voice, but eye opening or movement in response to physical stimulation
−5	No response to voice or physical stimulation

Table 2.3 **Delirium Detection Score**

Orientation
0—orientated to time, place, and personal identity, able to concentrate
1—not sure about time and/or place, not able to concentrate
4—not orientated to time and/or place
7—not orientated to time, place, and personal identity

Hallucinations
0—none
1—mild hallucinations at times
4—permanent mild-to-moderate hallucinations
7—permanent severe hallucinations

Agitation
0—normal activity
1—slightly higher activity
4—moderate restlessness
7—severe restlessness

Anxiety
0—no anxiety when resting
1—slight anxiety
4—moderate anxiety at times
7—acute panic attacks

Myoclonus/convulsions
0—none
1—myoclonus
7—convulsions

Paroxysmal sweating
0—no sweating
1—almost not detectable, only palms
4—beads of perspiration on the forehead
7—heavy sweating

Altered sleep–waking cycle
0—none
1—mild, patient complains about problems to sleep
4—patient sleeps only with high medication
7—patient does not sleep despite medication at night, tired at day time

Tremor
0—none
1—not visible, but can be felt
4—moderate tremor (arms stretched out)
7—severe tremor (without stretching arms)

Adapted from Luetz et al.[17]

Table 2.4 Confusion Assessment Method for the Intensive Care Unit (CAM-ICU)

Feature 1: Acute Onset or Fluctuating Course: Positive if you answer "yes" to either 1A *or* 1B.   Positive   Negative

   1A: Is the patient different from his/her baseline mental status?   Yes   No

   1B: Has the patient had any fluctuation in mental status in the past 24 h as evidenced by fluctuation on a sedation scale (e.g., RASS), Glasgow Coma Scale, or previous delirium assessment?

Feature 2: Inattention: Positive if score for either 2A or 2B is <8. Attempt the Attention Screening Examination (ASE) Letters first. If patient is able to perform this test and the score is clear, record the score and move to Feature 3. If patient is unable to perform this test or the score is unclear, perform the ASE Pictures. If you perform both tests, use the ASE Pictures results to score the Feature.   Positive   Negative

   2A: ASE Letters: Record score (enter "NT" for not tested). *Directions:* Say to the patient, *"I am going to read you a series of 10 letters. Whenever you hear the letter 'A,' indicate by squeezing my hand."* Read letters from the following letter list in a normal tone: S A V E A H A A R T. Scoring: Errors are counted when patient fails to squeeze on the letter 'A' and when the patient squeezes on any letter other than 'A.'   Score (out of 10): _____

   2B: ASE Pictures: Record score (enter "NT" for not tested). Directions are included on the picture packets.   Score (out of 10): _____

Feature 3: Disorganized Thinking. Positive if the combined score is <4.   Positive   Negative

   3A: Yes/No Questions: (Use either Set A or Set B; alternate on consecutive days if necessary):   Combined Score (3A + 3B): _____ (out of 5)

Set A	Set B
1. Will a stone float on water?	1. Will a leaf float on water?
2. Are there fish in the sea?	2. Are there elephants in the sea?
3. Does 1 pound weigh more 2 two pounds?	3. Do 2 pounds weigh more than 1 pound?
4. Can you use a hammer to pound a nail?	4. Can you use a hammer to cut wood?

Score_____ (Patient earns 1 point for each correct answer out of 4.)

3B: Command: *Directions:* Say to the patient, *"Hold up this many fingers"* (examiner holds two fingers in front of patient). *"Now do the same thing with the other hand"* (not repeating the number of fingers). If the patient is unable to move both arms, for the second part of the command, say to the patient, *"Add one more finger."*

Score_____ (Patient earns 1 point if able to successfully complete the entire command.) | Positive | Negative

Feature 4: Altered Level of Consciousness: Positive if the actual RASS score is anything other than "0" (zero). | Positive | Negative

Overall CAM-ICU: Add Features 1 and 2 and either Feature 3 or Feature 4.

RASS, Richmond Agitation Sedation Scale.
From Luetz et al.[17]

Table 2.5 **Neurologic Findings in Acutely Confused Patients in the Intensive Care Unit**

Diagnosis	Testing
Aphasia	Agrammatism
	Paraphasia
	Impaired naming
	Impaired writing
	Abnormal prosody
	Overuse of connectors (*if, and, but*)
	Neologisms
Apraxia	No weakness but no motor performance
	Inability to copy or pantomime
Abulia	Grasp, snout reflex
	Motor impersistence
	Paratonia (gegenhalten)
Agnosia	Neglect of left side
	Cortical blindness
	Prosopagnosia

In Practice

What should the neurologist think and do when approaching a delirious patient? It is not complicated: find a possible structural brain lesion, find a possible drug, find a possible drug that has been withdrawn, inquire about alcohol or drug abuse with close friends or family members, and suggest a more effective treatment (if possible). Most delirious patients have no acute structural lesion. Acute strokes— a nondominant hemispheric stroke—can cause severe agitation as a predominant sign. Some clinical signs are typically seen but may be less obvious to the non-neurologist. Remember that a patient with classic Wernicke encephalopathy rambles on, and many family members and even physicians would call it "agitation".

Drugs can cause delirium but we do not know how often. Known examples are opioids, corticosteroids, aluminum-containing antacids, β-adrenergic blockers, tacrolimus, cyclosporine, and histamine receptor antagonists. Perhaps most importantly, a history may be obtained from any available family member to establish (1) prior cognitive decline (one in three patients with dementia becomes delirious in the hospital), (2) alcohol use (many drink, and some drink a lot with family members who of course may deny that), and (3) prior psychiatric disorders or medications. Other risk factors are shown in Figure 2.2.

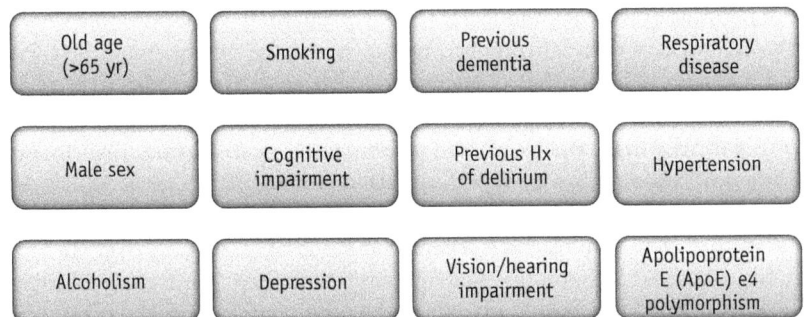

Figure 2.2 Risk factors predisposing for delirium.[15]

It seems well established, as a result of multiple cohort studies, that delirium is associated with increased mortality, prolonged ICU stay, and also cognitive impairment.[11,16] A comprehensive study found that patients with prolonged delirium are at higher risk for later cognitive impairment which can be severe and which can necessitate assistance with most daily tasks.[24] CT and magnetic resonance imaging (MRI) can be predictive. It is likely that those with subsequent cognitive impairment "had a running start." Delirium in a liver transplant recipient is more commonly seen when there is diffuse cortical atrophy, but this may also be related to the increased prevalence of liver transplantation for alcoholic cirrhosis.[6,20] White matter changes that are identified as leukoaraiosis on MRI also seem to predispose to delirium during an ICU stay, but none of these findings seems to predict prolonged cognitive decline.

The approach to ICU delirium or acute confusional state requires a new set of laboratory tests that may include a lumbar puncture, EEG, and new neuroimaging, but also should include a measurements of serum creatine kinase for neuroleptic malignant syndrome and serotonin syndrome, arterial blood gases, lactic acid, blood urea nitrogen, and serum ammonia concentration. Most of these studies may be superfluous, and even a new finding may not explain the sudden appearance of delirium.

TREATMENT OF DELIRIUM

Pharmacologic treatment of delirium should not include benzodiazepines unless there is a clear alcohol-withdrawal delirium or withdrawal from benzodiazepines. Antipsychotics are potentially concerning because they increase the risk of a prolonged QT interval and, with that, a risk of serious arrhythmias. Haloperidol is a traditional medication but has a poor safety profile when used as an intravenous (IV) infusion (tachyarrhythmias and torsades de pointes).[29,36]

Haloperidol blocks dopamine receptors throughout the brain, and it works on the assumption that delirium is caused by an excess of dopamine.[18,22] Its dose is 1–5 mg every 8 hours, but it may be used far more frequently, such as 5 mg every 2 hours IV until the patient is calm. Its half-life is long (on average, 15–20 hours), and the time to peak plasma concentration is 5–10 minutes; therefore, it is the quickest solution to severe agitation. Often, 30–45 minutes is needed before significant effects are seen. Side effects are clearly related to total dose, and some patients have received several hundreds of milligrams over the course of a day. Torsades de pointes evolving into sustained ventricular fibrillation requiring electroshock treatment is well known. Hypomagnesemia, hypocalcemia, and hypokalemia play a role and require correction before and after haloperidol administration. The risk of in-hospital neuroleptic malignant syndrome after haloperidol administration must be very low and very few neurologists with busy hospital practices have seen a single case. Use of haloperidol in patients with acute brain injury is still somewhat concerning, because several cases have been reported with worsening of the brain injury and resulting dopamine shortage. Data suggest that its use may reduce mortality, but the drug has largely been replaced by dexmedetomidine.[18,22]

Treatment options are summarized in Tables 2.6 and 2.7. The level of sedation can be titrated by using the Richmond Agitation Sedation Scale, which is a semiquantitative way of evaluating the adequacy of sedation.

Treatment should begin with trying to protect the patient. Physical restraints using wrist bands or gloves (Posey glove) to prevent the patient from grasping a line are very useful, but it is hard to prove that they reduce harm (or self-extubation) in daily practice, where constant restraint is never possible (i.e., a patient needs only a few seconds of free access to pull at a tube). Moreover, many patients who self-extubate do not need reintubation and may be telling the physician that they have been intubated too long. Restraint orders are driven by physicians but always require adequate documentation of their rationale. In some patients, they are really unavoidable; in others, they just cause more agitation (and higher doses of antipsychotics). Another "treatment" is the use of an around-the-clock sitter (family member or nurse aid), well-lit rooms

Table 2.6 **Treatment of Acute Confusion in the Intensive Care Unit**

- Eliminate trigger
- Stop benzodiazepines or anticholinergics
- IV dexmedetomidine** (0.2–0.7 mcg/kg/hour)
- IV haloperidol* (1–5 mg q8h)
- Quetiapine* (25–200 mg q12h)
- IV lorazepam** (2–4 mg/h)

*Increased dosing may cause concerning QT interval prolongation.
**Preferred for alcohol withdrawal.

Table 2.7 **Sedatives Commonly Used in the Intensive Care Unit**

Drug (trade name)	Mechanisms of action	Typical adult dose	Pharmacokinetic properties	Adverse effects
Midazolam (Versed)	$GABA_A$ agonist	Bolus, 1–5 mg; infusion, 1–5 mg/h	Half-life, 3–11 h; active metabolite accumulates with prolonged infusion; metabolized by hepatic oxidation, with renal excretion of active metabolite	Possibly a higher risk of delirium and tolerance than with certain other sedatives
Lorazepam (Ativan)	$GABA_A$ agonist	Bolus, 1–4 mg; infusion, 1–5 mg/h	Slower onset (5–20 min) than that of midazolam or diazepam (2–5 min); half-life, 8–15 h; metabolized by hepatic glucuronidation, with no active metabolites, so offset may be more predictable than that of midazolam in critical illness	Possibly a higher risk of delirium and tolerance than with certain other sedatives
Propofol (Diprivan)	$GABA_A$ agonist, with other effects, including on glutamate and cannabinoid receptors	50–200 mg/h or 1–3 mg/kg/h	Half-life, 30–60 min after infusion; longer after prolonged infusion because of redistribution from fat stores; metabolized by haptic glucuronidation and hydroxylation	Vasodilatation or negative inotropy causing hypotension or bradycardia; propofol infusion syndrome (lactic acidosis, arrhythmia, and cardiac arrest), mostly associated with prolonged infusion rates of greater than 4–5 mg/kg/h; hypertriglyceridemia; pancreatitis

* $GABA_A$, γ-aminobutyric acid type A.
From Reade and Finfer.[30]

with clocks, and familiar objects (e.g., home blanket, photographs)—but the benefit of all of this is unknown.

Other, less tested options include promotion of sleep, assuming a relation between sleep deprivation and delirium. Music therapy (music through headphones) has not proved useful in delirium but reduces anxiety when compared with noise-cancelling headphones.[22,25,30]

The next line of action is to discontinue any benzodiazepine and, if feasible, corticosteroids.[3,23,31,32] The best treatment for agitated delirium remains IV dexmedetomidine. Because bolus, or loading, of dexmedetomidine can cause hypotension, administration of the initial dexmedetomidine bolus might best be avoided. Early hypotension is often used as a reason not to administer dexmedetomidine and can preclude the administration of this very effective treatment for delirium. Hypotension without bradycardia responds very well to a fluid bolus during the beginning of the infusion. (Preexisting hypovolemia is a common contributing factor.) Bradycardia is clearly a reason not to continue dexmedetomidine. Dexmedetomidine prolongs the QT interval (>450 msec), but major cardiac arrhythmias are unusual. The hemodynamic effect of dexmedetomidine may be biphasic, with initial hypertension (vasoconstriction peripherally) and later hypotension. Rapid infusion of the loading dose (<10 minutes) is a common cause for hypotension.

Patients with liver function abnormalities need a dosage reduction, but the typical infusion dose is 0.2–0.7 mg/kg/h (usually starting at 0.4 mg/kg/h). More delirium-free days and fewer ventilator days were associated with the use of dexmedetomidine when compared with lorazepam. Alternative choices are quetiapine 50–200 mg every 12 hours, but it works much more slowly (12–24 hours) and is better for waxing and waning agitation.[13] Quetiapine is thus less useful in severe agitation and when there is a need for quick resolution.

Putting It All Together

- There is a definitional tangle of "delirium" with "acute confusion."
- Drowsiness is not hypoactive delirium.
- Agitated delirium requires multiple treatment approaches.
- ICU tools for nursing staff to recognize delirium are available and helpful.
- Delirium in the ICU is linked to later risk for cognitive difficulties and dementia.
- IV medication first—other measures (restraints, noise and visit reduction) later.

By the Way

- Most patients with confusion are not examined by neurologists.
- Pain may significantly "drive" confusion.
- Benzodiazepines are overused, particularly the long-lasting ones.
- Dexmedetomidine is preferred in any type of delirium.
- Benzodiazepines or dexmedetomidine are preferred in alcohol withdrawal delirium.
- Sedation may add additional $500 to daily ICU costs.

> **Acute Confusion by the Numbers**
> - ~70% of mechanically ventilated patients may become "delirious".
> - ~40% of patients with delirium are detected by ICU screening tools.
> - ~20% of patients are delirious on their first or second ICU day.
> - ~10% of patients may have an identifiable reason for delirium.
> - ~5% of patients may still develop delirium after leaving ICU.

References

1. Aguirre GK, D'Esposito M. Topographical disorientation: a synthesis and taxonomy. *Brain* 1999;122:1613-1628.
2. Banh HL. Management of delirium in adult critically ill patients: an overview. *J Pharm Pharm Sci* 2012;15:499-509.
3. Barr J, Fraser GL, Puntillo K, et al. Clinical practice guidelines for the management of pain, agitation, and delirium in adult patients in the intensive care unit. *Crit Care Med* 2013;41:263-306.
4. Brown CH. Delirium in the cardiac surgical ICU. *Curr Opin Anaesthesiol* 2014;27:117-122.
5. Brummel NE, Jackson JC, Pandharipande PP, et al. Delirium in the ICU and subsequent long-term disability among survivors of mechanical ventilation. *Crit Care Med* 2014;42:369-377.
6. Buis CI, Wiesner RH, Krom RA, Kremers WK, Wijdicks EF. Acute confusional state following liver transplantation for alcoholic liver disease. *Neurology* 2002;59:601-605.
7. Devinsky O, D'Esposito M. *Neurology of Cognitive and Behavioral Disorders*. Oxford, England: Oxford University Press, 2004.
8. Ely EW, Inouye SK, Bernard GR, et al. Delirium in mechanically ventilated patients: validity and reliability of the Confusion Assessment Method for the Intensive Care Unit (CAM-ICU). *JAMA* 2001;286:2703-2710.
9. Ely EW, Margolin R, Francis J, et al. Evaluation of delirium in critically ill patients: validation of the Confusion Assessment Method for the Intensive Care Unit (CAM-ICU). *Crit Care Med* 2001;29:1370-1379.
10. Ely EW, Shintani A, Truman B, et al. Delirium as a predictor of mortality in mechanically ventilated patients in the intensive care unit. *JAMA* 2004;291:1753-1762.
11. Flannery AH, Flynn JD. More questions than answers in ICU delirium: pressing issues for future research. *Ann Pharmacother* 2013;47:1558-1561.
12. Fraser GL, Gagnon DJ, Riker RR. SLEAP: A wake-up call to question the oversimplification of ICU delirium. *Crit Care Med* 2015;43:703-705.
13. Hawkins SB, Bucklin M, Muzyk AJ. Quetiapine for the treatment of delirium. *J Hosp Med* 2013;8:215-220.
14. Hoy SM, Keating GM. Dexmedetomidine: a review of its use for sedation in mechanically ventilated patients in an intensive care setting and for procedural sedation. *Drugs* 2011;71:1481-1501.
15. Janz DR, Abel TW, Jackson JC, et al. Brain autopsy findings in intensive care unit patients previously suffering from delirium: a pilot study. *J Crit Care* 2010;25:538e537-538e512.
16. Lorenzo M, Aldecoa C, Rico J. Delirium in the critically ill patient. *Trends Anaesth Crit Care* 2013;3:257-264.
17. Luetz A, Heymann A, Radtke FM, et al. Different assessment tools for intensive care unit delirium: which score to use? *Crit Care Med* 2010;38:409-418.
18. Milbrandt EB, Kersten A, Kong L, et al. Haloperidol use is associated with lower hospital mortality in mechanically ventilated patients. *Crit Care Med* 2005;33:226-229.

19. Moore RD, Bone LR, Geller G, et al. Prevalence, detection, and treatment of alcoholism in hospitalized patients. *JAMA* 1989;261:403–407.
20. Ouimet S, Kavanagh BP, Gottfried SB, Skrobik Y. Incidence, risk factors and consequences of ICU delirium. *Intensive Care Med* 2007;33:66–73.
21. Ouimet S, Riker R, Bergeron N, et al. Subsyndromal delirium in the ICU: evidence for a disease spectrum. *Intensive Care Med* 2007;33:1007–1013.
22. Page VJ, Ely EW, Gates S, et al. Effect of intravenous haloperidol on the duration of delirium and coma in critically ill patients (Hope-ICU): a randomised, double-blind, placebo-controlled trial. *Lancet Respir Med* 2013;1:515–523.
23. Pandharipande P, Shintani A, Peterson J, et al. Lorazepam is an independent risk factor for transitioning to delirium in intensive care unit patients. *Anesthesiology* 2006;104:21–26.
24. Pandharipande PP, Girard TD, Jackson JC, et al. Long-term cognitive impairment after critical illness. *N Engl J Med* 2013;369:1306–1316.
25. Peitz GJ, Balas MC, Olsen KM, Pun BT, Ely EW. Top 10 myths regarding sedation and delirium in the ICU. *Crit Care Med* 2013;41:S46–S56.
26. Pisani MA, Kong SY, Kasl SV, et al. Days of delirium are associated with 1-year mortality in an older intensive care unit population. *Am J Respir Crit Care Med* 2009;180:1092–1097.
27. Pun BT, Ely EW. The importance of diagnosing and managing ICU delirium. *Chest* 2007;132:624–636.
28. Radtke FM, Franck M, Schust S, et al. A comparison of three scores to screen for delirium on the surgical ward. *World J Surg* 2010;34:487–494.
29. Rea RS, Battistone S, Fong JJ, Devlin JW. Atypical antipsychotics versus haloperidol for treatment of delirium in acutely ill patients. *Pharmacotherapy* 2007;27:588–594.
30. Reade MC, Finfer S. Sedation and delirium in the intensive care unit. *N Engl J Med* 2014;370:444–454.
31. Schreiber MP, Colantuoni E, Bienvenu OJ, et al. Corticosteroids and Transition to Delirium in Patients With Acute Lung Injury. *Crit Care Med* 2014;42:1480–1486.
32. Shadvar K, Baastani F, Mahmoodpoor A, Bilehjani E. Evaluation of the prevalence and risk factors of delirium in cardiac surgery ICU. *J Cardiovasc Thorac Res* 2013;5:157–161.
33. Spronk PE, Riekerk B, Hofhuis J, Rommes JH. Occurrence of delirium is severely underestimated in the ICU during daily care. *Intensive Care Med* 2009;35:1276–1280.
34. Trzepacz PT. Is there a final common neural pathway in delirium? Focus on acetylcholine and dopamine. *Semin Clin Neuropsychiatry* 2000;5:132–148.
35. Vocat R, Staub F, Stroppini T, Vuilleumier P. Anosognosia for hemiplegia: a clinical-anatomical prospective study. *Brain* 2010;133:3578–3597.
36. Wang HR, Woo YS, Bahk WM. Atypical antipsychotics in the treatment of delirium. *Psychiatry Clin Neurosci* 2013;67:323–331.
37. Wolters AE, van Dijk D, Pasma W, et al. Long-term outcome of delirium during intensive care unit stay in survivors of critical illness: a prospective cohort study. *Crit Care* 2014;18:R125.
38. Zaal IJ, Slooter AJ. Delirium in critically ill patients: epidemiology, pathophysiology, diagnosis and management. *Drugs* 2012;72:1457–1471.

3

Encephalopathies of Organ Dysfunction

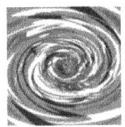

Organ dysfunction could affect neuronal and astroglial functions. This may occur when indispensable substrate is not provided (oxygen and glucose), when serum electrolytes are out of normal range (abnormal natremias), or when new toxic intermediates circulate (glutamine). Although it has traditionally been thought that improving organ function leads to improved neuronal function, this is not always the case. An additional challenge for neurologists is to explain to unconvinced intensivists that markedly improving organ function may lead to delayed neurologic improvement. Moreover, the "toxic-metabolic encephalopathy" of yesterday may now turn out to be posterior reversible encephalopathy syndrome (PRES) in uremia, brain edema in fulminant hepatic failure, and leukoencephalopathy in thyroiditis. On occasion, a patient's rapid decline in consciousness with acute kidney injury is caused by a newly diagnosed thrombotic thrombocytopenic purpura requiring effective plasma exchange.

Multiorgan dysfunction is common in medical and surgical intensive care units and often part of a sepsis syndrome. In sepsis, the most commonly affected organs are the lungs, kidneys, and liver, and damage is usually linked to marked hypotension. Thus, the brain is also an "innocent bystander" in shock, and an immediate abnormality of cerebral blood flow (CBF) may not be compensated for and lead to ischemic changes in the most vulnerable watershed zones.

This chapter attempts to clarify the neurologic complications of acute organ failure causing or caused by critical illness. Important questions are the following: How does acute renal failure or liver failure contribute to the clinical picture? When and why is hypotension associated with distributive shock deleterious to the brain? What is the main driver in septic encephalopathy? When do structural abnormalities explain the clinical findings in acute metabolic derangement?

There is a steady number of consults requesting the evaluation of patients for neurologic injury resulting from organ injury. Encephalopathies associated with organ failure comprise a sprawling number of disorders, and neurologists are pointedly aware that it is difficult to be certain what is going on in the brain and with the patient.

Principles

This section discusses the pathophysiologic mechanisms that lead to the clinical manifestations of acute organ failure and the characteristic findings for each organ.

ACUTE PULMONARY DISEASE

Regardless of its cause, respiratory failure leads to insufficient oxygen supply and retention of carbon dioxide. Hypercarbia causes a respiratory acidosis. This hypercapnic acidosis (assuming no chronically retained carbon dioxide and resetting of respiratory modulators) causes irritability followed by drowsiness and, eventually, "CO_2 narcosis." Patients have small (miotic) pupils, as seen in opioid intoxication and any deep sleep. Hypercapnic acidosis also may result in some multifocal myoclonus and asterixis, but usually when the arterial partial pressure of carbon dioxide ($PaCO_2$) is greater than 70 mm Hg. Hypercapnic acidosis is clearly related to oxygen administration and usually produces the higher levels of hypercapnia seen in a hypoventilating patient ($PaCO_2$ rarely rises substantially without oxygen administration).

The only treatment for hypercapnic acidosis is mechanical ventilation, and settings can normalize oxygen administration and normalize hypercarbia to a certain level (permissive hypercarbia). Such return to normal values results often in impressive clinical improvement and return to awareness and alertness. Cortical depression or dampened neuronal activity—using electroencephalography as a marker—has been repeatedly shown with hypercapnia. In addition, with hypercapnia there is an increase in CBF that increases tissue oxygenation. This vascular response in the brain is an adaptive response to tissue acidosis. Increased CBF also increases intracranial pressure (ICP). (It is estimated that each 1 mm Hg increase in $PaCO_2$ is accompanied by a 5% increase in CBF.) In general, CBF is less sensitive to hypoxemia, and it will remain constant until a severe hypoxemia is reached (Figure 3.1).

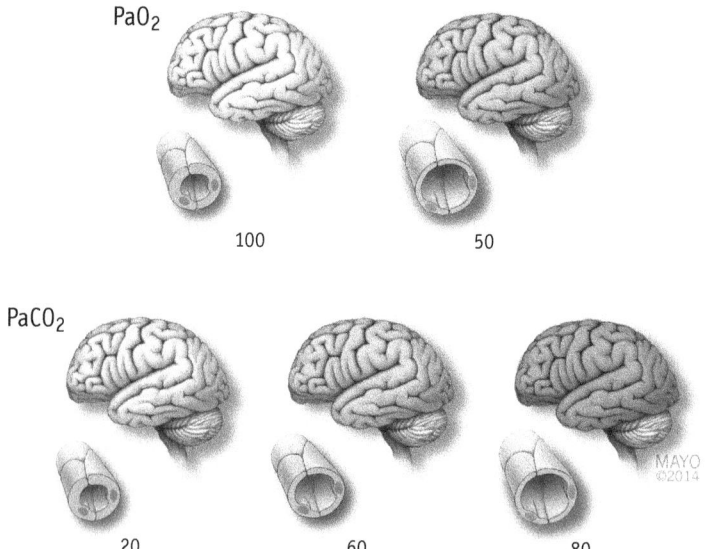

Figure 3.1 Relation between cerebral blood flow and the partial pressures of oxygen (PaO_2) and carbon dioxide ($PaCO_2$). Shading indicates degree of cerebral blood flow (decreased in right brain image, normal in middle brain image, and increased in left brain image) with corresponding PaO_2 and $PaCO_2$ values.

Hypoxemia can cause neuronal injury, although not if circulation is maintained. A very low PaO_2 (<30 mm Hg) is needed to result in syncope. A vagal response and hypotension from reduced right ventricular filling and reduced cardiac output is a possible operative mechanism. Only in extreme asphyxia does the accompanying hypotension damage the brain. This mechanism also plays a role in tissue hypoxemia due to carbon monoxide poisoning. Lesions are often seen in the globus pallidus because of its vulnerability as a watershed area.[28]

When ischemia occurs, there is exposure to the excitatory neurotransmitter glutamate and opening of the calcium and sodium channels. The increased calcium level initiates an apoptosis pathway and also accelerates lipid degradation and increases intercellular free fatty acids. The cytoskeleton proteins autolyze as a result of activation of calcium-dependent proteinases, and this activates the initial steps of apoptosis (for further discussion, see another volume in this series, *Recognizing Acute Brain Injury*).

ACUTE RENAL FAILURE

Acute renal failure causes a number of so-called uremic retention solutes. Each has the potential to increase the permeability of the blood–brain barrier and impair cellular transport mechanisms. It has been known for a number of years that guanidine compounds are increased in patients with uremia, particularly in the cerebrospinal fluid (CSF). Other relevant compounds are likely to be present in severely uremic patients. In addition, glutamate is released and binds to the *N*-methyl-D-aspartate (NMDA) and α-amino-3-hydroxy-5-methyl-4-isoxazolepropionic acid (AMPA) receptors. These are all major neurotoxins that can cause the manifestations seen with acute renal disease.[7,29-32] There is also some evidence that uremic encephalopathy is associated with the release of inflammatory markers that result in the upregulation of inflammatory processes and leads to disruption of microvascular barriers. Hypercoagulability is also seen in patients with chronic end-stage renal disease as a result of changes in coagulation, fibrinolysis, and platelet functions and may eventually lead to cerebral infarctions. What complicates matters is that there is a poor relationship between simple laboratory tests (e.g., urea, creatinine) and neurologic manifestations.

Uremic encephalopathy usually produces impaired wakefulness, failure to sustain attention, and, eventually, restlessness, dysarthria, and even development of an agitated delirium. Patients with severe uremic encephalopathy develop asterixis. Asterixis is a lapse of posture that, when frequent, can very much look like tremors. It is more prevalent in drowsy patients and disappears after the first round of dialysis. Some nephrologists doubt a correlation between encephalopathy and certain creatinine and blood urea nitrogen values, but use asterixis, among other markers, to indicate the need for dialysis.

What has become clear over the years is that PRES is a major manifestation of acute end-stage renal disease. Mostly, PRES is related to major flare-ups of hypertension or new presentations of severe hypertension, but it can present in the absence of this relationship. It is typically recognized as a decreased level of consciousness, but the patient may have transient cortical blindness and seizures or simply an acute confusional syndrome. The diagnosis is typically made by magnetic resonance imaging (MRI) (i.e., fluid-attenuated inversion recovery and diffusion-weighted imaging [DWI] sequences), although computed tomography scans can show early hypodensities in the posterior brain regions. (Often these abnormalities either are not recognized or are misinterpreted as early infarctions.)

As alluded to earlier, PRES is a major manifestation in intensive care units in patients who are hypertensive or have a sepsis syndrome. It reflects vasogenic edema in the white matter caused by leaky arteries. The most frequent location is parietooccipital, but it can occur in thalami and in posterior fossa structures. Hemorrhage into the areas of vasogenic edema occurs in 10%–20% of cases and there may be mild subarachnoid hemorrhage. Restricted diffusion on MRI DWI may occur and may not always be associated with later clinical findings on follow-up, but when it involves large areas, it reflects permanent cerebral infarction. PRES can be expected with a sudden surge of hypertension, poor kidney function, autoimmune disease, and evolving gram-positive sepsis.[17,40] In any unexplained "altered mental status" in a patient with advanced kidney disease (with or without hypertensive urgency), it is important to consider PRES and to pursue the diagnosis.

Dialysis complications are now unusual, and other conditions are far more likely (e.g., subdural hematoma).[6,27] Rapid dialysis may produce an acute syndrome that nowadays is seldom seen. There are two schools of thought. In the "reverse urea" hypothesis,[35,41–43] a significant urea gradient between blood and brain after dialysis results in water influx to the brain. In normal circumstances, urea diffuses more slowly than water across the blood–brain barrier; when blood urea is rapidly increased, an osmotic difference is created, resulting in water extraction from the brain. Reversing this gradient with dialysis results in a higher urea concentration in the brain compared with plasma, and this phenomenon causes brain edema. Naturally, it can be corrected by adding urea or mannitol or by increasing the sodium concentration of the dialysate.[41–43] The "idiogenic osmole" hypothesis[2,3] argues that the urea concentrations in the brain are not high enough to account for the increase in brain water. Brain swelling, in this view, is promoted by the formation of idiogenic osmoles, possibly organic acids produced during rapid dialysis, which lead to an increase in brain osmolality and water influx. Direct measurements showed an increase in brain osmolality that could not be explained by the sum of urea and electrolyte concentrations, suggesting a new formation of osmotically active particles (osmoles). Formation of organic osmoles in the brain during such osmotic stress has been documented.

ACUTE LIVER FAILURE

Staying on the same subject, even more substances have been investigated in acute liver failure. The real challenge is to prove that these intermediates are part of an organized process or pathway. The significance of these factors, alone or in combination, and whether they should represent avenues for potential pharmaceutical intervention, remains uncertain but definitively interesting. The list seems endless, but it is of interest to review some of the proposed mechanisms.

Ammonia plays an important role, and it is a consistent clinical observation that patients rarely develop hepatic encephalopathy with an arterial ammonia concentration of less than 75 mmol/L. It is known by pathologists that most of the abnormalities are seen where the ammonia burden is greatest—areas with higher blood supply such as the brain, basal ganglia, cerebellum, and cortex. Manganese has also been found, with active deposition in the globus pallidus, substantia nigra, and thalami. Increased manganese can also be identified as hyperintense signal on T1-weighted images on MRI.

Ammonia has been implicated in the pathogenesis of hepatic encephalopathy, perhaps through an imbalance between inhibitory and excitatory neurotransmitters. The γ-aminobutyric acid (GABA) neurotransmitter system, an inhibitory system, possibly plays a prominent role. GABA causes hyperpolarization of neuronal membrane through opening of chloride channels and influx of chloride into the cells. It has been observed in animal models that hepatic encephalopathy has many similarities to encephalopathy induced by drugs that potentiate GABA action. It appears that the degree of hepatic encephalopathy is correlated with CSF levels of GABA. Furthermore, flumazenil, a benzodiazepine antagonist, has been shown to improve the encephalopathy, at least in some cases. These findings have led to the suggestion that endogenous substances with benzodiazepine-like properties contribute to the neuropsychiatric manifestations of hepatic encephalopathy.[21]

Other possible explanations of the mechanism of hepatic encephalopathy are controversial. Mercaptans, short-chain fatty acids, and depletion of neurotransmitters (e.g., norepinephrine, dopamine) have been implicated. Ammonia also impairs postsynaptic inhibition in cortex, thalamus, and brainstem; interferes with chloride outward pumping; decreases (excitatory) glutaminergic synaptic function; increases 5-hydroxytryptamine degradation by monoamine oxidase; and increases dopamine metabolites, such as homovanillic acid and 3-methoxytyramine—but all that information has no clinical relevance.

What is notably different and urgent is that acute liver failure is associated with the development of cerebral edema in the worst cases.[26,37,46] In contrast, in many patients who develop chronic liver failure (e.g., portosystemic encephalopathy), the development of symptoms is far more gradual and may have a different origin. Portosystemic encephalopathy associated with acute liver disease is a consequence of cirrhosis and an indirect result of increased blood ammonia levels.

Cerebral edema in fulminant acute liver failure became recognized in the early 1960s, and hepatologists saw mostly massive tonsillar herniation at autopsy, although it was initially dismissed by neurologists as likely clinically irrelevant. Hepatologists and liver transplantation surgeons observed that patients with clinically suspected brain edema responded well to high doses of osmotic agents. When cerebral edema also became apparent on computed tomography scans and ICP monitors recorded increased ICP, it became a target for management. Patients could be salvaged if ICP was adequately controlled until a new liver was implanted and functional.

The pathophysiology of the brain in patients with acute liver necrosis is thus different from chronic progressive liver damage, and there are multiple pathophysiologic mechanisms that play a role. One is a deficit in the ability of astrocytes to take up glutamate from the excess cellular space. That, in itself, leads to excitotoxicity of the neuronal glutamate receptors. Aquaporin-4, which is involved in brain water transport, may also play a role. In many situations, the abnormalities are a result of alterations in cerebral hemodynamics, which may be initiated by the production of nitric oxide.

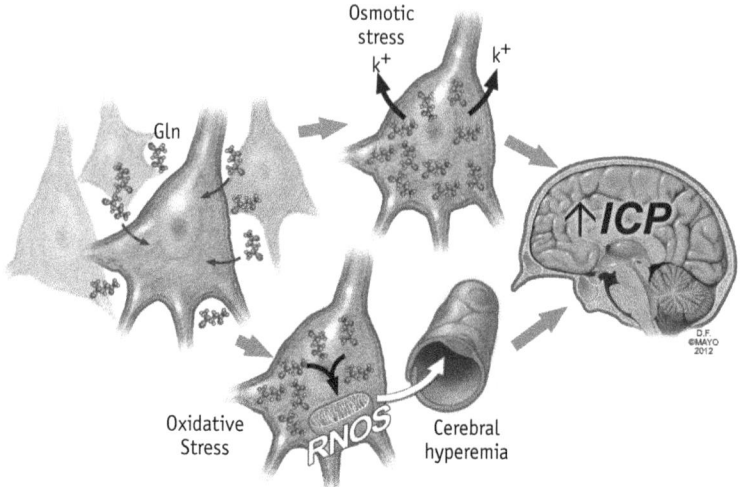

Figure 3.2 Pathways and mechanisms of liver failure leading to increased ICP. Gln, glutamine; ICP, intracranial pressure; RNOS, reactive nitrogen oxide species.

Increased nitric oxide and CBF may be important in the development of cerebral edema and intracranial hypertension. Ammonia is detoxified by astrocytes through the synthesis of glutamine, and this may act as an osmolyte. Astrocyte swelling then leads to the formation of reactive oxygen and reactive nitrogen oxide species, and eventually to apoptosis (Figure 3.2).[9,12]

ACUTE PANCREATIC DISEASE

The stress of critical illness causes hyperglycemia, but seldom at levels that generate neurologic symptoms. However, existing diabetes can become deranged, leading to a nonketotic hyperosmolar state. Sepsis, corticosteroids, or a high dose of dopamine may provoke such a dysregulation. Coma or stupor requires a five- to tenfold increase in serum glucose, and values should reach 600–800 mg/dL. Plasma osmolality (often in the range of 350 mOsm/L) correlates better with the decrease in level of consciousness. Focal neurologic findings are common and often trigger consults for alleged stroke. Focal seizures may occur. Patients may be aphasic and may have marked asymmetries, all of which disappear with serum glucose correction. Rehydration with small doses of insulin will be required. More common is an acute pancreatitis, but shock and acute respiratory distress syndrome rapidly become part of the picture. In more severely affected patients, acute renal failure ensues, causing additional problems and a very mixed picture.[16,45] There is no determinable "pancreatic encephalopathy."

ACUTE THYROID FAILURE

Thyroid hormone has an effect on cerebral neuronal activity, but the triiodothyronine receptors are concentrated more in the limbic system and amygdala than in the brainstem. Both reduced and increased brain metabolism have been reported in hypothyroid and hyperthyroid patients subjected to positron emission tomography, but these findings correlate with depression and anxiety, not new neurologic symptomatology. Other major confounders are hyponatremia (which initially causes muscle cramps) and hypoglycemia. Much less often, a pituitary mass or hypothalamic tumor is the primary cause of thyroid dysfunction, and its mass effect can cause impaired consciousness. Pituitary apoplexy may be a cause of hypothyroidism, but more commonly it leads to secondary adrenocorticotropic hormone deficiency.

Hashimoto's encephalopathy is recognized as a pathologically defined entity involving perivascular, nonvasculitic, lymphocytic infiltration in brain, meninges, cortex, basal ganglia, thalami, and hippocampus. This rare disorder can be difficult to detect, because thyroid function may be clinically and biochemically normal. It has also been known under more explanatory names: steroid-responsive encephalopathy associated with autoimmune thyroiditis and nonvasculitic autoimmune meningoencephalitis. The laboratory findings include increased or high-normal serum thyrotropin levels and increased thyroid peroxidase antibodies.

Thyroid dysfunction has a great impact on neuromuscular function, but the effects are mostly gradual and mild. Occasionally, a thyrotoxic myopathy of sufficient severity is encountered. I have seen a patient with Graves' disease (free thyroxine levels increased fivefold) who had an iodine contrast study followed by a severe and prolonged (4 months) flaccid paralysis with facial diplegia and hypophonia, even after thyroid markers were corrected. Muscle pain as a result of rhabdomyolysis in this setting is common.[10,13]

ACUTE ADRENAL DISEASE

Acute adrenal insufficiency (Addison's disease) is a potential problem in any intensive care unit. Adrenal crisis typically occurs in patients previously treated with corticosteroids in whom the dose was not increased during infection or was abruptly withdrawn.

Clinically, patients are in shock and often hypoglycemic, and a seizure may have occurred. Some patients become markedly delirious. A morning cortisol level of less than 3 mcg/dL (80 nmol/L) is a good screening method when cortisol peaks at the stress of awakeing, but the electrolyte abnormalities point in the right direction. Chronic Addison's disease results in pigmentations, but these are not present in previously treated patients. Addison's disease is manifested by rapidly evolving shock and dehydration. Laboratory diagnosis reveals the triad of hyponatremia, hyperglycemia, and hyperkalemia. Hypercalcemia may occur and may be sufficiently severe to decrease responsiveness. Weakness in a patient with Addisonian crisis may be associated with hyperkalemic myopathy and flaccid tetraplegia or, in exceptional cases, with a Guillain-Barré–like syndrome.

The encephalopathy of adrenal insufficiency may have features of profound perceptual impairment, with lethargy progressing to coma. Bilateral papilledema has been described in early terminal cases, but only in association with pathologically demonstrated cerebral edema.

Replenishment with corticosteroids and replacement of the sodium and water deficit and electrolytes are the mainstays of treatment for Addisonian crisis.

MULTIORGAN FAILURE

The most common cause for multiorgan failure in the intensive care unit is sepsis. How sepsis can lead to a "septic brain" remains poorly understood. One theory is that the presence of peripheral cytokines may cause alterations in the blood–brain barrier or, through other pathways, microglial activation. This will lead to the production of reactive oxygen species and neuronal dropout. Sepsis and septic shock are often also understood as a systemic inflammatory reaction syndrome (SIRS). SIRS has been diagnosed when two of the following five symptoms are present: hyperthermia or hypothermia, tachycardia, tachypnea, leukocytosis, and leukopenia, but recent studies found this condition may not be easily recognizable. Sepsis expresses tissue factor, disturbs coagulation, produces capillary clots, and reduces tissue perfusion, causing lungs, liver, kidneys, or brain to fail. Bacteria create endotoxins (e.g., lipopolysaccharide [LPS]) that activate cells producing inflammatory cytokines such as interleukin 6, interleukin 1, and tumor necrosis factor. However, these endotoxins cross the blood–brain barrier only if there is impairment.[19,20,36] We know little of what happens in the brain, and the progress made in understanding inflammation processes may not translate to brain injury.

Blood–brain permeability may be impaired due to increased nitric oxide synthase in endothelial cells. Prolonged exposure to LPS reduces excitability of hippocampal cells[38] and causes cell loss. Sepsis models have typically used cecal ligation and puncture, but the brain has been inadequately studied.[1,22] Sepsis may also affect hypothalamic neuroendocrine systems (e.g., oxytocin), and thus a connection with the limbic system exists through which encephalopathy could be explained.[39] Current concepts include systemic inflammation resulting in the disruption of the blood–brain barrier and neuronal injury from complement proteins, cytokines, and nitric oxide. Brain injury and its manifestations often occur before obvious multiorgan failure, but in clinical practice, they cannot be distinguished. Impaired cerebrovascular autoregulation has been found and has been correlated with encephalopathy.[8,11,14,15,18]

Patients in septic shock may have bacterial meningitis as their primary disorder; this should be recognized, because the antibiotics used for sepsis may not penetrate CSF well enough, and adjustment will be needed.

In Practice

It is assumed that, in most situations, patients will have acute brain dysfunction from sepsis-associated encephalopathy or from new-onset acute renal or liver failure. PRES is so prevalent that it should always be considered and actively investigated. Neurologists for many years had the tendency to call it all "multifactorial metabolic encephalopathy" and then list the abnormalities that made up the patient's critical illness. Nothing could be more unhelpful.

The task at hand is to summarize clinical findings and to obtain comprehensive neuroimaging in most cases. The fundamentals here are to isolate the main driver of neurologic manifestations, to see if neurologic examination changes after correction, and if not to consider other possible explanations, such as structural injury.

One of the most difficult derangements to assess clinically is hypoxemia and hypercarbia. The effects of worsening hypercarbia (and lesser extent hypoxemia) on performance and clarity of thought are substantial, particularly if the patient has increased work of breathing due to a developing acute lung injury. After intubation, sedation will be confounding, and it will be difficult to assess cognition.

Septic encephalopathy is difficult to distinguish from other metabolic disturbances that could involve hypercapnia, fever, acute renal or hepatic encephalopathy, and, in some situations, acute hyperglycemia. Under any circumstance, septic encephalopathy should be considered only after a central nervous system infection, alcohol or drug intoxication, Wernicke's encephalopathy, nonconvulsive status epilepticus, serotonin syndrome, neuroleptic malignant syndrome, and immune-mediated encephalitis have been excluded.

One approach to patients who have been septic and have diminished responsiveness is to minimize and discontinue sedatives and analgesics, eliminate reversible causes (beginning with the most likely ones), and continue the search for an associated condition. Because fever is prominent, septic encephalopathy can be mimicked by serotonin syndrome, in which the patient has marked hyperreflexia, rigidity, and dysautonomia; each of these symptoms can be easily treated by discontinuation of serotonergic agents, control of fever, and aggressive treatment with benzodiazepines and cyproheptadine. Occasionally, cefepime neurotoxicity is recognized and the patient will improve after cefepime has been replaced by an alternative antimicrobial drug.

Hepatic encephalopathy has been categorized in clinical stages of stepwise worsening (Table 3.1). The description of each stage varies somewhat in the literature, but the differences between adjacent stages are clear enough to be helpful in clinical practice. Problems arise with the more severe stages, in which more neurologic differentiation is needed—in particular, assessment of brainstem reflexes and breathing patterns. Partial loss of brainstem reflexes, need for intubation, and failure to track horizontally are important components of the Full Outline of UnResponsiveness (FOUR) score and therefore are useful additions for grading of hepatic encephalopathy with reduced scores predicting in-hospital mortality.[34]

Treatment of hepatic encephalopathy consists of lactulose administration and correction of precipitants (e.g., gastrointestinal bleeding, infection, high protein intake). If there is no improvement, rifaximin[5,46] or neomycin is added. If this is unsuccessful, one should evaluate the patient for portosystemic shunt[25,33] or therapy using the Molecular Adsorbent Recirculating System (MARS, Gambro)[4] (Figure 3.3). In MARS, a membrane that is impermeable to proteins but capable of exchanging water-soluble and protein-bound toxins and a recycled protein containing dialysate are used.[44] A meta-analysis of studies using MARS did show some but not significant survival benefit in patients with liver failure

Table 3.1 **Grades of Hepatic Encephalopathy**

Grade	Impairment		SONIC criteria
	Intellectual	Neuromuscular	
0	Normal	Normal	Normal
	Normal examination findings; subtle changes in work or driving	Minor abnormalities of visual perception or on psychometric or number tests	Covert
1	Personality changes, attention deficits, irritability, depressed state	Tremor and incoordination	Covert
2	Changes in sleep–wake cycle, lethargy, mood and behavioral changes, cognitive dysfunction	Asterixis, ataxic gait, speech abnormalities (slow and slurred)	Overt
3	Altered level of consciousness (somnolence), confusion, disorientation, amnesia	Muscular rigidity, nystagmus, clonus, Babinski's sign, hyporeflexia	Overt
4	Stupor and coma	Oculocephalic reflex increased, unresponsiveness to noxious stimuli	Overt

SONIC, spectrum of neurocognitive impairment in cirrhosis.

From Leise et al.[26]

when compared with standard medical therapy.[24] More observational studies are needed to define the role of MARS in the treatment of these disorders.

ICP monitoring is recommended for patients with the higher (3 and 4) hepatic encephalopathy, in centers with expertise in ICP monitoring, and for patients awaiting and undergoing liver transplantation. Complications (e.g., hemorrhage) during ICP monitor placement occur in 5%–10% of patients (Figure 3-4). This may be prevented

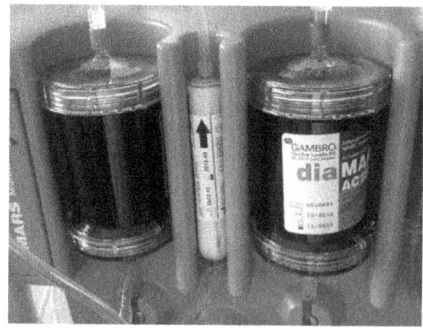

Figure 3.3 The Molecular Adsorbent Recirculating System (MARS).

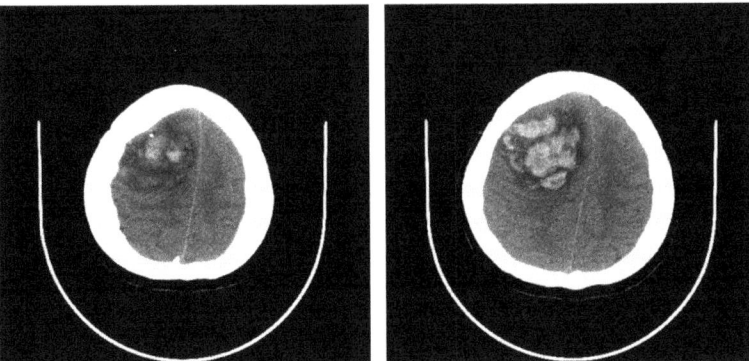

Figure 3.4 Computed tomography scan of parenchymal hemorrhage associated with intracranial pressure monitor (note white dot) in a patient with fulminant hepatic failure.

by the use of fresh-frozen plasma and prothrombin complex concentrate during ICP monitor placement, but whether later aggressive correction of international normalized ratio and platelets is needed is not exactly known (most parenchymal hemorrhages we have seen were noted after an asymptomatic interval suggesting ongoing intervention might be needed). Treatment of cerebral edema follows traditional methods of ICP management. Any underlying factors that could worsen the ICP, such as agitation, coughing, frequent turning, endotracheal suctioning, and severe hypertension, need to be minimized.

Vasoconstriction induced by hypocapnia can decrease regional CBF and inflict secondary ischemic brain injury. Increasing evidence suggests that hypocapnia can induce substantial adverse effects including cardiac arrhythmias, myocardial ischemia, and bronchospasm. Therefore, therapeutic hypocapnia should usually be limited to emergency management of life-threatening increases in ICP.

The choice of mannitol or hypertonic saline depends on the clinical situation. The serum sodium level has to be monitored when hyperosmolar therapy is used. It is generally accepted that hypertonic saline should not be used if the serum sodium level is greater than 160 mEq/L. Several uncontrolled studies have suggested effective control of brain edema and intracranial hypertension with the induction of hypothermia. A recent study group[23] found that using hypothermia in 97 patients did not improve overall and transplant free survival. Barbiturates are an option in cases resistant to hyperosmolar therapy. Barbiturate clearance is (expectedly) markedly reduced in patients with acute liver failure, and when administered, this will preclude neurologic assessment for prolonged periods, making it a much less attractive option for treatment of intracranial hypertension. As a very last resort, thiopental is commonly given as a 4 mg/kg loading dose followed by infusion starting at 1 mg/kg/h, with gradual upward titration until ICP control is established or hypotension develops. ICP monitoring is usually started at about the time of intubation for worsening encephalopathy and should be continued at least 1 or 2 days after liver transplantation. Usually, patients undergo grafting within 3 days of hospitalization, because the window of opportunity is small.

Putting It All Together

- Metabolic encephalopathy may involve structural lesions.
- Acute fulminant hepatic failure causes brain edema and increased ICP that can be effectively treated only with liver transplantation.
- PRES is common in acute or chronic kidney disease.
- Acute thyroid or adrenal disease is very rare.
- Acute pancreatitis causes brain injury from hyperglycemia, shock, and hypoxemia

---

By the Way

- Endocrinopathies in critical illness rarely manifest neurologically.
- Organ dysfunction results in poor clearance of sedatives and analgesics.
- Dialysis quickly improves uremia and the patient's alertness.
- Dialysis has virtually no neurologic manifestations not already caused by renal disease.

Organ Dysfunction by the Numbers

- ~50% of patients with cirrhosis have hepatic encephalopathy.
- ~30% of patients with sepsis have encephalopathy.
- ~25% of patients with acute renal failure may develop PRES.
- ~5% of patients remain comatose after septic shock.
- ~3% of patients with severe renal disease develop acute subdural hematoma.

References

1. Ari I, Kafa IM, Kurt MA. Perimicrovascular edema in the frontal cortex in a rat model of intraperitoneal sepsis. *Exp Neurol* 2006;198:242–249.
2. Arieff AI. More on the dialysis disequilibrium syndrome. *West J Med* 1989;151:74–76.
3. Arieff AI, Massry SG, Barrientos A, Kleeman CR. Brain water and electrolyte metabolism in uremia: effects of slow and rapid hemodialysis. *Kidney Int* 1973;4:177–187.
4. Banares R, Nevens F, Larsen FS, et al. Extracorporeal albumin dialysis with the molecular adsorbent recirculating system in acute-on-chronic liver failure: the RELIEF trial. *Hepatology* 2013;57:1153–1162.
5. Bass NM, Mullen KD, Sanyal A, et al. Rifaximin treatment in hepatic encephalopathy. *N Engl J Med* 2010;362:1071–1081.
6. Bechar M, Lakke JP, van der Hem GK, Beks JW, Penning L. Subdural hematoma during long-term hemodialysis. *Arch Neurol* 1972;26:513–516.
7. Biasioli S, D'Andrea G, Feriani M, et al. Uremic encephalopathy: an updating. *Clin Nephrol* 1986;25:57–63.

8. Bolton CF, Young GB, Zochodne DW. The neurological complications of sepsis. *Ann Neurol* 1993;33:94–100.
9. Cordoba J, Garcia-Martinez R, Simon-Talero M. Hyponatremic and hepatic encephalopathies: similarities, differences and coexistence. *Metab Brain Dis* 2010;25:73–80.
10. Couillard P, Wijdicks EF. Flaccid quadriplegia due to thyrotoxic myopathy. *Neurocrit Care* 2014;20:296–297.
11. d'Avila JC, Santiago AP, Amancio RT, et al. Sepsis induces brain mitochondrial dysfunction. *Crit Care Med* 2008;36:1925–1932.
12. Dhiman RK, Kurmi R, Thumburu KK, et al. Diagnosis and prognostic significance of minimal hepatic encephalopathy in patients with cirrhosis of liver. *Dig Dis Sci* 2010; 55:2381–2390.
13. Duyff RF, Van den Bosch J, Laman DM, van Loon BJ, Linssen WH. Neuromuscular findings in thyroid dysfunction: a prospective clinical and electrodiagnostic study. *J Neurol Neurosurg Psychiatry* 2000;68:750–755.
14. Eidelman LA, Putterman D, Putterman C, Sprung CL. The spectrum of septic encephalopathy: definitions, etiologies, and mortalities. *JAMA* 1996;275:470–473.
15. Gofton TE, Young GB. Sepsis-associated encephalopathy. *Nat Rev Neurol* 2012;8:557–566.
16. Greer SE, Burchard KW. Acute pancreatitis and critical illness: a pancreatic tale of hypoperfusion and inflammation. *Chest* 2009;136:1413–1419.
17. Hefzy HM, Bartynski WS, Boardman JF, Lacomis D. Hemorrhage in posterior reversible encephalopathy syndrome: imaging and clinical features. *Am J Neuroradiol* 2009;30:1371–1379.
18. Iacobone E, Bailly-Salin J, Polito A, et al. Sepsis-associated encephalopathy and its differential diagnosis. *Crit Care Med* 2009;37:S331–S336.
19. Jacob A, Brorson JR, Alexander JJ. Septic encephalopathy: inflammation in man and mouse. *Neurochem Int* 2011;58:472–476.
20. Jacob A, Hensley LK, Safratowich BD, Quigg RJ, Alexander JJ. The role of the complement cascade in endotoxin-induced septic encephalopathy. *Lab Invest* 2007;87:1186–1194.
21. Jones EA, Skolnick P, Gammal SH, Basile AS, Mullen KD. The gamma-aminobutyric acid A (GABAA) receptor complex and hepatic encephalopathy: some recent advances. National Institutes of Health conference. *Ann Intern Med* 1989;110:532–546.
22. Kafa IM, Bakirci S, Uysal M, Kurt MA. Alterations in the brain electrical activity in a rat model of sepsis-associated encephalopathy. *Brain Res* 2010;1354:217–226.
23. Karvellas CJ, Stravitz RT, Battenhouse H. et al. Therapeutic hypothermia in acute liver failure: a multicenter retrospective cohort analysis. *Liver Transplant* 2015;21:4–12.
24. Khuroo MS, Farahat KL. Molecular adsorbent recirculating system for acute and acute-on-chronic liver failure: a meta-analysis. *Liver Transpl* 2004;10:1099–1106.
25. Laleman W, Simon-Talero M, Maleux G, et al. Embolization of large spontaneous portosystemic shunts for refractory hepatic encephalopathy: a multicenter survey on safety and efficacy. *Hepatology* 2013;57:2448–2457.
26. Leise MD, Poterucha JJ, Kamath PS, Kim WR. Management of hepatic encephalopathy in the hospital. *Mayo Clin Proc* 2014;89:241–253.
27. Leonard A, Shapiro FL. Subdural hematoma in regularly hemodialyzed patients. *Ann Intern Med* 1975;82:650–658.
28. Lo CP, Chen SY, Lee KW, et al. Brain injury after acute carbon monoxide poisoning: early and late complications. *Am J Roentgenol* 2007;189:W205–W211.
29. Locke S, Merrill JP, Tyler HR. Neurologic complications of acute uremia. *Arch Intern Med* 1961;108:519–530.
30. Lockwood AH. Metabolic encephalopathies: opportunities and challenges. *J Cereb Blood Flow Metab* 1987;7:523–526.
31. Lockwood AH. Neurologic complications of renal disease. *Neurol Clin* 1989;7:617–627.
32. Mahoney CA, Arieff AI. Uremic encephalopathies: clinical, biochemical, and experimental features. *Am J Kidney Dis* 1982;2:324–336.
33. Mitzner SR. Extracorporeal liver support: albumin dialysis with the Molecular Adsorbent Recirculating System (MARS). *Ann Hepatol* 2011;10 Suppl 1:S21–S28.

34. Mouri S, Tripon S, Rudler M, et al. FOUR Score, a reliable score for assessing overt hepatic encephalopathy in cirrhotic patients. *Neurocrit Care* 2015;22:251–257.
35. Pappius HM, Oh JH, Dossetor JB. The effects of rapid hemodialysis on brain tissues and cerebrospinal fluid of dogs. *Can J Physiol Pharmacol* 1967;45:129–147.
36. Pinheiro da Silva F, Machado MC, Velasco IT. Neuropeptides in sepsis: from brain pathology to systemic inflammation. *Peptides* 2013;44:135–138.
37. Scott TR, Kronsten VT, Hughes RD, Shawcross DL. Pathophysiology of cerebral oedema in acute liver failure. *World J Gastroenterol* 2013;19:9240–9255.
38. Semmler A, Widmann CN, Okulla T, et al. Persistent cognitive impairment, hippocampal atrophy and EEG changes in sepsis survivors. *J Neurol Neurosurg Psychiatry* 2013;84:62–69.
39. Sendemir E, Kafa IM, Schafer HH, Jirikowski GF. Altered oxytocinergic hypothalamus systems in sepsis. *J Chem Neuroanat* 2013;52:44–48.
40. Sharma A, Whitesell RT, Moran KJ. Imaging pattern of intracranial hemorrhage in the setting of posterior reversible encephalopathy syndrome. *Neuroradiology* 2010;52:855–863.
41. Silver SM. Cerebral edema after hemodialysis: the "reverse urea effect" lives. *Int J Artif Organs* 1998;21:247–250.
42. Silver SM. Cerebral edema after rapid dialysis is not caused by an increase in brain organic osmolytes. *J Am Soc Nephrol* 1995;6:1600–1606.
43. Silver SM, Sterns RH, Halperin ML. Brain swelling after dialysis: old urea or new osmoles? *Am J Kidney Dis* 1996;28:1–13.
44. Stange J. Extracorporeal liver support. *Organogenesis* 2011;7:64–73.
45. Wada K, Takada T, Hirata K, et al. Treatment strategy for acute pancreatitis. *J Hepatobiliary Pancreat Sci* 2010;17:79–86.
46. Williams R, James OF, Warnes TW, Morgan MY. Evaluation of the efficacy and safety of rifaximin in the treatment of hepatic encephalopathy: a double-blind, randomized, dose-finding multi-centre study. *Eur J Gastroenterol Hepatol* 2000;12:203–208.

4

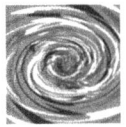

The Postoperative Cardiac Patient

Cardiac surgery often involves a coronary artery bypass graft (CABG) procedure, valve replacement, or valve repair, and each of these operations requires cardiopulmonary bypass. Valve surgery is an open-heart surgery and offers more potential for complications than CABG. It is reconstructive, performed mostly to repair a valve affected by degenerative disease or, more dramatically, a valve destroyed by bacterial endocarditis. Usually after cardiopulmonary bypass, there is a smooth transition to heart function, but management of hemodynamics with inotropic therapy may be needed. In many cases, all goes well and the patient benefits greatly. Neurologists are not often seen in cardiovascular units, which admit thousands of postoperative patients each year. According to the American Heart Association, an estimated 100,000 cardiac valve surgeries are performed annually in the United States.

It may be surprising that neurologic complications are uncommon, and neurologists have always assumed that many complications go undetected. Illustratively, when a neurologist examined all patients pre- and postoperatively, stroke occurred in an unexpectedly high 17% and was the highest reported incidence in the literature.[22] In older patients with increasing comorbidity factors, one can expect more acute neurology consults after cardiac surgery.

When asked to evaluate a patient with a possible new neurologic symptom, the consulting neurologist is typically not fully aware of the hemodynamic threats or other major problems that have occurred during cardiac surgery. On entering the cardiac intensive care unit (ICU), the neurologist might find the patient being treated with extracorporeal membrane oxygenation (ECMO), a balloon pump, or a combination of inotropic and sedative drugs. It may sometimes seem impossible to judge whether the patient's condition represents a true new neurologic problem or an expected slow transition to full awakening after a major surgical procedure with intraoperative complications.

Therefore, acute calls to the neurologist to see a patient who has undergone a major cardiovascular procedure often relate to newly perceived major asymmetries in limb function, new-onset seizure, failure to awaken after several days of weaning from sedatives and analgesics, and possible peripheral nerve injury. The immediate question a surgeon asks is, "How do I know whether the patient is still sedated or has had a major brain injury?" The immediate questions that the consulting neurologist should ask are the following: Am I able to adequately assess the patient, knowing that a large amount of opioids have been used during surgery? Are the focal findings the result of a central or a peripheral injury of the nervous system? Is neuroimaging available, and if not, can it be obtained in this critically ill patient? Does the patient need treatment for a single seizure? How helpful is magnetic resonance imaging (MRI), knowing that the patient likely will have multiple small infarcts as a result of the procedure?

These are important immediate considerations when consulting on a postoperative cardiac patient. Some patients develop a florid delirium because cardiac surgery is a good enough stressor, and there is a fairly high prevalence (Chapter 2). However, most problems after cardiac surgery come later, when the patient is home and family members start noticing poor decisions, ceaseless memory lapses, and sometimes even an inability to be safe when not supervised.[14,28,29] These patients with prolonged difficulties are rarely seen by neurologists, and they have never taken ownership of them.

Principles

Cardiovascular surgery is a major surgical procedure for several reasons. The events and their possible mechanisms are shown in Table 4.1. But this surgical specialty is also changing and minimally invasive techniques have been developed for cardiac surgery,

Table 4.1 **Potential Mechanisms of Neurologic Complications After Cardiac Surgery**

Neurologic complication	Potential mechanism
Hypoxic-ischemic encephalopathy	Acute low cardiac output, hypotension, shock, hypoglycemia
Ischemic and hemorrhagic stroke	Thromboemboli
Pituitary apoplexy	Proposed mechanisms: factors related to the extracorporeal bypass, anticoagulation, low cerebral blood flow, anesthetic agents, presence of subclinical pituitary tumor
Seizure	Drug toxicity, tranexamic acid, cerebral thromboembolism, cerebral air embolism
Ischemic infarction of the brain or spinal cord	Thromboembolism, air embolism, vessel trauma, hypotension, underlying coagulopathy related to use of intra-aortic balloon pump.
Encephalopathy	Sedatives, analgesics, showers of microemboli
Visual loss	Optic nerve ischemia, retinal artery embolism
Horner's syndrome	Injury to the cervical sympathetic chain
Brachial plexopathy	Stretching, direct trauma or compression
Phrenic nerve injury	Stretching, direct trauma, ischemia or topical hypothermia

including common coronary bypass and valve surgery. These techniques include mini-sternotomy and small thoracotomy for access to the mitral valve or aortic valve. Percutaneous aortic valve replacement with fluoroscopic imaging has become a common intervention. Transmyocardial laser revascularization creates channels through a left thoracotomy incision or standard sternotomy. These channels direct blood into the myocardium from the ventricle, resulting in significant relief of angina. Cardiac arrhythmias are the most expected complications. Vaporization of myocardium may generate left ventricular bubbles.

One core principle for the neurologist is therefore that some description of common and current cardiac surgical procedures is needed. What is it that the cardiac surgeons do? Where do they insert catheters? What do they clamp? What lesions do they potentially create? Equally important is the management by anesthesiologists and if they encountered problems.

Major cardiac surgery involves cardiopulmonary bypass. CABG is most frequently performed on a beating heart without on-pump cardiopulmonary bypass. This reduces and eliminates cross-clamping of the aorta, which can be related to serious injuries to the central nervous system (CNS). Bubble expansion and air embolism during the cooling phase of the bypass, hypotension, and increased intracranial pressure resulting from obstruction of the vena cava cannula have all been observed during cardiopulmonary bypass, and these risks disappear if it is not used. However, most centers continue to use cardiopulmonary bypass.

The device is shown in Figure 4.1. In principle, venous blood passes through an oxygenator and returns to the ascending aorta. A large catheter is placed, which

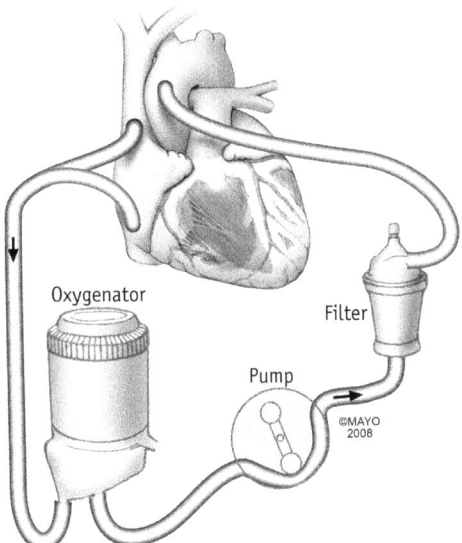

Figure 4.1 Setup of cardiopulmonary bypass device. (See Chapter 6 for information on extracorporeal membrane oxygenation, which is a similar concept but with different cannula placement.)

in itself could induce emboli. Atheromatous debris can be dislodged and has been identified during continuous transcranial Doppler ultrasound monitoring. These emboli manifest as additional high-frequency sounds superimposed on a silent band created by the known pulsatile flow of the bypass. Embolic events also have been associated with refilling of the heart in a later stage of the procedure. Important clinical trials have compared off-pump with on-pump CABG, and no differences in long-term outcome (1 year) pertaining to the quality of life or neurocognitive function were found, as assessed by a multiple batteries of tests. This finding has resulted in a reemphasis on the patient's prior risk factors as possible causes of postoperative problems—such risk factors include prior carotid artery disease and atherosclerotic disease of the aorta.

Several perfusion-related problems may occur, but all of what follows is uncommon or even exceptionally rare. First, aortic cannulation problems may cause any of the following: (1) excessive carotid flow if the cannula is too long and close to the carotid artery, (2) hypoperfused carotid artery if the angle of the cannula is misdirected, and (3) a high-velocity jet ("sandblast") against the atherosclerotic artery if the cannula is too small (it can embolize material or even occlude the vessel as a result of intimal dissection).

Malposition of the arterial cannula can cause aortic dissection. Usually, this is detected if the pressure in the aortic cannula does not match the systemic pressure. The left radial arterial catheter has a low pressure, and the right radial arterial catheter has a high pressure.

Sudden reduced venous drainage may occur, and the reservoir level will be low, requiring large volumes of fluids before venous drainage is restored. Large air bubbles due to lifting of the heart by the surgeon have been implicated. Gas embolism may occur because of a defective or clotted oxygenator and can be a cause of postoperative stroke. Massive gas embolism is very rare but may require hyperbaric oxygen treatment and a retrograde perfusion protocol. Inadequate anticoagulation may lead to visual observation of clot in the oxygenator. After removal of the cardiopulmonary bypass, a cardiovascular decompensation may occur. This left ventricular failure requires inotropic drug administration, often a combination of drugs (milrinone with phenylephrine, dopamine, or dobutamine). In some of these patients, ECMO support may have to be resumed to avoid cardiovascular collapse.

Anesthesia changes during the procedure, and some anesthesiologists use the bispectral index to assess the depth of anesthesia.[20] Opioids or benzodiazepines may be administered, increase in the depth of anesthesia during major surgical manipulation may occur, and many patients are given propofol during rewarming. Neuromuscular blockade to prevent shivering is often used, and these levels may be affected by temperature changes, blood loss, and cardiac function. Many patients develop hyperglycemia as a result of surgical stressors. Inotropes also stimulates glycogenolysis, and glucose-containing solutions may contribute greatly. Aggressive control is recognized, but with more aggressive control of hyperglycemia, hypoglycemia is a serious risk. It is important to anticipate that glucose levels that are trending down require very frequent checks and "unsuspected hypoglycemia" may occur soon after surgery. Blood transfusions to correct a low hematocrit remain an unresolved controversy. Relative anemia may be a factor if other parameters (oxygenation) are abnormal. Both may well result in compromised cerebral blood flow and oxygen requirements. The effect of hypothermia on cerebral blood flow and cerebral metabolism has been well studied and it produces marked metabolic suppression.[5,20,24]

So when a stroke occurs, what could be the mechanism—watershed infarctions from hypoperfusion or emboli? There continues to be an understanding that hypoperfusion may play an important role in the development of neurologic injury, and this may be particularly relevant for patients with long-standing hypertension, in whom prolonged hypotension could jeopardize areas at risk. In these strictly autoregulated areas (regulated upward due to chronic hypertension), a mild hypotension is sufficient to cause marginal to poor perfusion. Surgeries that include clamping of the aorta increase the embolization risk, and avoidance or modification of techniques continues to be an important and possible preventive measure. The "no touch" technique is an area of debate among cardiac surgeons.[16]

The question is whether revisitation of the blood pressure tracings during surgery provides useful information for the consulting neurologist. Marked drops in blood pressure, and even brief periods of cardiopulmonary resuscitation, may not necessarily increase the risk of postoperative complications.[1] In fact, a link between intraoperative hypotension and postoperative outcome has never consistently been established or proven.

Retrospective analyses of large cardiac surgery trials, even in patients randomized to mean arterial blood pressures (MAPs) of 80–100 mm Hg versus 50–60 mm Hg, found no differences in neurologic complications in those patients with higher MAPs.[4] However, the definitions of stroke and neurologic complications were poorly detailed. Others have found that systolic blood pressure variability is related to a higher risk of mortality, but again with no clear relationship to stroke incidents. Some have suggested that a MAP higher than 80 mm Hg reduces neurologic complications in cardiac surgery, but supporting evidence is lacking.[21]

In general, the complexity of surgery does relate to the risk of ischemic stroke, with a rapid increase if CABG is combined with valvular surgery, if CABG is associated with unilateral or bilateral carotid stenosis, or if surgery involves aortic repair or double- or triple-valve surgery. Double- or triple-valve surgery can increase the risk of stroke fivefold. Questions designed to elicit the risk factors for perioperative stroke during on-pump CABG are summarized in Table 4.2.

An important preoperative question has been whether intraoperative monitoring with various devices (e.g., infrared spectroscopy, transcranial Doppler ultrasound) increases the recognition of cardioembolic events. None of the studies has been definitive and there is not sufficient data to show that cerebral monitoring improves outcome.[20] The interest in transcranial Doppler monitoring for emboli has waned.[26] Intraoperative monitoring with cerebral near-infrared spectroscopy may be useful, but there are insufficient data to clearly link the results with events during surgery.[8,36]

Another major principle is to not overinterpret neuroimaging. MRI after cardiac surgery often shows multiple fluid-attenuated inversion recovery imaging

Table 4.2 **Questions to Staff Concerning Patients in the Intensive Care Unit with Impaired Consciousness**

Nursing staff or attending consultant
• Intraoperative cardiopulmonary resuscitation? • Intraoperative shock? • Presence of an asymptomatic interval after surgery? • Current hypotension requiring vasopressors? • Hypoxemia requiring a high level of positive end-expiratory pressure? • Total amount of analgesics and sedatives infused? • Myoclonus, eye deviation, eyelid blinking?

abnormalities.[17] Several diffusion-weighted imaging (DWI) lesions may also be found, and these "silent infarctions" are often seen in asymptomatic patients. The more extensive these lesions are, the more severe cognitive impairment is found. However, the data are conflicting. In certain situations, findings may be related to a preoperative coronary angiogram rather than surgery. Several studies have found silent MRI lesions in about one of every three patients who underwent MRI after surgery,[31] and even higher in a recent prospective study with half of the patients showing lesions.[22]

There is also sufficient evidence that prior cardiac surgery is not a risk factor for a long-standing cognitive impairment or later development of dementia. Mild brain edema may be seen on postoperative computed tomography (CT) scans. It is diffusely distributed but usually asymptomatic, and it is completely reversible. MRI (DWI with apparent diffusion coefficient mapping) is useful in excluding ischemic infarction as the cause of these changes. Cerebral swelling after CABG is assumed to represent a variant of hyperperfusion syndrome or reversible posterior encephalopathy syndrome. Sudden forced dilation of cerebral arteries may breach the blood–brain barrier and cause extravasation of fluid with resulting edema.

Another unclear situation is whether atrial fibrillation is associated with increased stroke risk. Several studies have found that about half of patients develop atrial fibrillation after CABG and that this is related to later postoperative stroke.[2,3,11,32,36] Aggressive control of atrial fibrillation with the use of β-blockade, magnesium, amiodarone, statins, atrial pacing, or even posterior pericardiotomy has not been able to reduce postoperative stroke rates despite successful reduction of atrial fibrillation.[21]

Efforts to reduce postoperative ischemic injury have included hypothermic cardiac arrest when the cerebral metabolic rate for oxygen is correlated with temperature. The cerebral metabolic rate is about 50% at 30°C, 25% at 20°C, and 10% at 10°C. This significantly lengthens the safety of ischemic time, from 5 to 45 minutes with deep hypothermia (10°C). Clinically, it appears that 30 minutes may be tolerated without significant cognitive deficits.[6,24]

In Practice

When does a cardiac surgeon decide that the patient has failed to awaken after a cardiovascular repair? Most patients have received large doses of fentanyl and benzodiazepines and may still be on a comparatively high dose. The likely anticipation is that when these drugs are discontinued, the patient will gradually become more responsive and when such improvement does not occur overnight and the next afternoon, the neurologist is called in. Neurologic consultation may also be triggered by a CT scan that shows new infarctions. Failure to awaken after surgery is likely less alarming than assumed, and one can expect that many patients take several days to awaken after a complex procedure. CT scans often show irrelevant or small abnormalities that cannot be attributed to a declining level of consciousness. It remains uncommon to find a permanently comatose patient, and in such cases, the circumstances are quite clear—something out of the ordinary has happened. When patients remain deeply comatose with abnormal motor responses CT scan can be diagnostic (Figure 4.2).[10]

Multiple vascular infarctions are almost always linked to severe aortic atherosclerotic disease (most cardiovascular surgeons would comment on such a finding) and

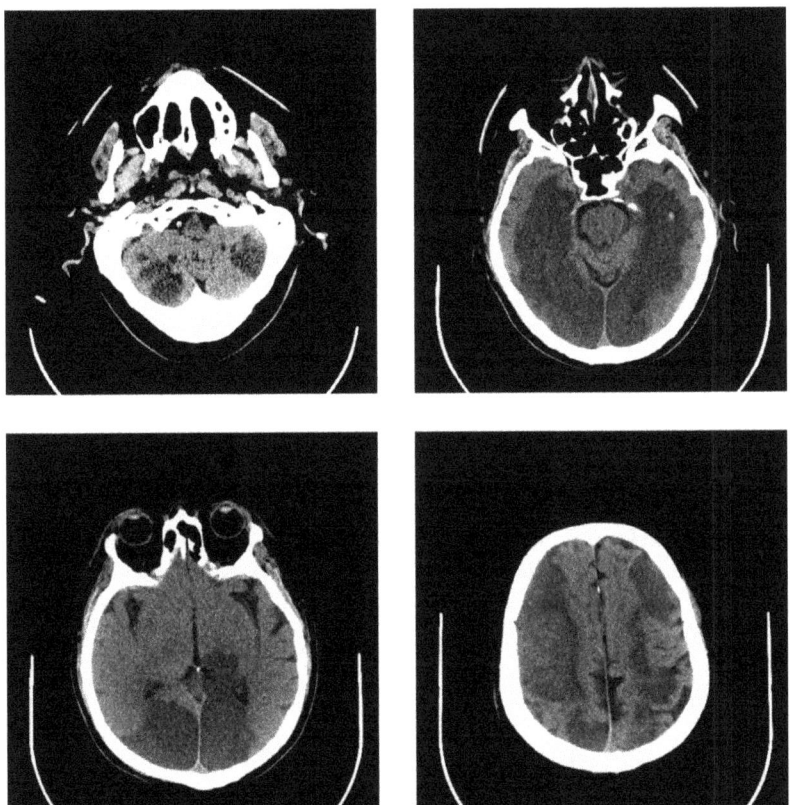

Figure 4.2 Computed tomography scan of a devastating postoperative stroke.

to embolization. Cardiac arrest occurring intraoperatively (or in the recovery room), hypotension, and use of ECMO may all cause diffuse cortical necrosis, which is easily visualized on MRI. Air emboli are very uncommon and are seen on CT causing abnormal "black spots." (These result from a bypass malfunction and not from a failure of the surgeon to appropriately de-air.)

I have seen an embolus to the basilar artery after cardiac surgery as a cause of postoperative coma, and the condition was recognized by pupil anisocoria, skew deviation, ocular bobbing, and extensor posturing—a constellation of signs that is hard to miss. Postoperative hypoglycemia (from overly aggressive insulin infusion) and hyponatremia (from overly aggressive free water use) should be considered. In any event, postoperative coma with widespread MRI abnormalities predict a very poor outcome, and most of these patients die from withdrawal of support or are discharged to a nursing home. Patients who have had cardiopulmonary arrest and remain comatose as a result of anoxic-ischemic injury could potentially be candidates for hypothermia. However, there is no experience on the pros and cons of this procedure, and most studies have found no significant improvement after therapeutic hypothermia in hospital stroke. For now, aggressive temperature management might be more feasible than hypothermia.

Seizures may also be a presenting symptom. They occur in a relatively small percentage of patients and typically are of the generalized tonic–clonic type, rarely partial. Patients who have postoperative seizures have a fivefold higher mortality rate than patients who do not, and seizures are often associated with large territorial infarcts and watershed infarcts. An association with antifibrinolytic agents has been found, but only with high doses of tranexamic acid and with renal failure.[9,13,15,18] Most cardiac surgeons use antifibrinolytic agents to prevent postoperative bleeding. Inhibition of fibrinolysis has been shown to reduce bleeding in various clinical situations associated with activation and dysregulation of the fibrinolytic pathway, including cardiac surgery. Whether a similar risk is present with high doses of aminocaproic acid (both are lysine analogs) is not known. The assumption is that tranexamic acid may have a direct neuronal excitatory effect because it can cross the blood–brain barrier—in animal experiments, direct cortical application caused seizures.[28] One could also postulate that the drug may cause more clotting and thus transiently increase the risk of cortical strokes and seizures. Seizures as a result of use of this drug occur just hours after surgery and when patient has been moved from the recovery room to the ICU. To prove correlation with these drugs, an MRI may be needed to exclude an ischemic stroke as a cause of seizures. Postoperative intracranial hemorrhage as a cause for seizures is rare and was found in only 8% of cases in one study.[9]

It is well established that seizures are more often seen in patients who have multiorgan failure; this includes renal failure, sepsis, and prolonged mechanical ventilation. Nonetheless, a seizure after cardiopulmonary surgery is an important clinical sign that indicates a structural injury to the brain, and therefore an MRI scan might be warranted to detect a new abnormality.[25] As alluded to earlier, small scattered DWI lesions may not necessarily be correlated and larger territorial infarcts need to be found to prove the association.

Although the incidence of seizures remains low, clinicians should target their approach based on whether the seizures are focal or generalized and on a review of history and medications. Seizures can be managed acutely with benzodiazepines.

Special concerns in this setting regarding the side-effect profile of antiepileptics that induce hepatic enzymes have led to the use of valproic acid and levetiracetam as worthwhile alternatives. Seizures are best briefly treated with levetiracetam (1,000 mg twice daily) or valproate (30 mg/kg IV loading dose, followed by 20 mg/kg maintenance dose divided into two doses). There is no rationale to treat beyond 4 weeks, and the drug can be tapered if electroencephalography is not showing an epileptic focus.

Cardiac surgery may also occur in a setting of infectious endocarditis, which poses new and complex problems.[27] The decision to proceed with valve replacement in a patient who has infective aortic or mitral endocarditis is usually related to the development of valve regurgitation and cardiac failure, but may also be related to ongoing embolization to the brain or other territories. The large doses of IV heparin used during cardiopulmonary bypass puts these patients at a higher risk for intracranial hemorrhage.[23] Most cardiovascular surgeons are concerned about hemorrhagic transformation of infarcts due to septic emboli. Stroke is not a contraindication for surgery; in fact, it is an indication for surgery.[34] Risk factors for septic emboli are endocarditis of the mitral valve, vegetation size (>10 mm), and pathogen (*Staphylococcus aureus*), but not the type of valve (native valve versus mechanical prosthetic valve replacement).[23] Many surgeons either wait 72 hours or opt for a 4-week delay in patients with infectious endocarditis.

These surgeries in endocarditis are generally far more problematic, with approximately 25% mortality from sepsis and a 50% survival rate in patients with endocarditis and cerebral emboli. Cerebral emboli are more commonly found when emboli have been documented in the spleen or kidney (mostly on CT of the abdomen). It remains very unclear whether early antibiotic therapy can prevent embolization, and some have argued that the best approach is mainly source control (meaning valve replacement in the case of a mobile vegetation). Moreover, whether a preoperative cerebral angiogram is needed is unresolved. Documentation of an unruptured mycotic aneurysm gives the surgeon pause. In endocarditis, approximately 10% of patients have mycotic aneurysm, and if there has been a cerebral hemorrhage, the incidence doubles to 20% (detection remains poor).[12] Finding a mycotic aneurysm may lead to coil occlusion but it is not certain if this prevents postoperative intracerebral hemorrhage (estimated 2%) from other leaking vasculitic arteries.

An acute ischemic stroke may be detected in the postoperative ICU. Nonetheless, the detection of acute new focal findings remains problematic and is often delayed, and therefore stroke onset remains unclear in many patients. In addition, thrombolytic agents cannot be used because of a substantial risk of thoracic bleeding or even the development of pericardiac hematoma. Therefore, the best approach would be to immediately proceed with CT angiography and CT perfusion. The CT perfusion is able to detect an established infarct or a possibility of salvaging areas (see another volume in this series, *Handling Difficult Situations*). If a large viable area is seen in a proximal stenosis, endovascular devices should be able to retrieve the embolus, with an opportunity for recovery. Some successful cases have been reported but the experience is very limited, and in many situations, acute stroke is detected late or there has been no recognized urgency.

Many patients and families are concerned about long-term effects, but this is not always addressed in preoperative discussion. Several earlier studies showed an immediate risk of cognitive dysfunction in a considerable proportion of patients. The risk is increased after valvular repair, particularly in older patients, but long-term outcome is more favorable than anticipated. Some recent studies have shown only a small proportion of patients with cognitive difficulties 3 months after valvular surgery.[7] One convincing review found little evidence of dementia after cardiac surgery.[33] There is also the possibility that cardiac surgery simply exacerbates a prior (not recognized) minimal cognitive impairment. No evidence exists that cardiac surgery directly causes progressive dementia.

There are several other highly unusual complications that may trigger a consult. Infarction of the spinal cord typically affects the midthoracic spinal cord level, between the circulatory areas of the descending spinal arteries and the artery of Adamkiewicz. Possible causes of spinal cord ischemia include the use of an intraaortic balloon pump (IABP), aortic trauma secondary to cross-clamping or insertion of an IABP, aortoiliac occlusive disease, microembolization of atherosclerotic plaques or cholesterol emboli, and major hypotension. Recognition and management are discussed in Chapter 5.

Peripheral injury may occur with faulty positioning, and retractors can cause injury, which is mostly reversible. The most common nerve injured in cardiac surgery is the lower trunk of the brachial plexus. Other nerves that may be damaged include the ulnar nerve, the recurrent laryngeal nerve, the saphenous nerve, the common peroneal nerve, and the cervical sympathetic chain. Brachial plexopathy may occur if the brachial plexus is stretched during a median sternotomy by the use of sternal retractors. Patients with injured nerves tend to be older and to have had longer operation times. The cervical sympathetic chain, which lies medial to the inferior trunk of the brachial plexus, may be injured during sternal retraction and may manifest as a Horner syndrome.

The saphenous nerve may be injured during harvesting of the long saphenous vein, resulting in anesthesia, hyperesthesia, and pain in the distribution of the saphenous nerve. In about 0.2% of patients, the common peroneal nerve is affected during CABG, with damage to the nerve at the fibular head due to nerve ischemia from compression or stretching. Although the severity of mononeuropathies after cardiac surgery can range from mild transient sensory neuropathy to disabling paralysis, symptoms almost always completely resolve.

Finally, the IABP is a mechanical device that was initially used for patients with perioperative cardiac failure and is now also used for those with pre-shock, severe congestive heart failure, or refractory angina. Significant neurologic deficits in one or both legs, ranging from a foot drop to almost total paralysis, have been associated with the use of IABP. In these patients, IABP insertion was via the femoral artery, and the neurologic deficits were hypothesized to be caused by the obstruction of blood flow or thromboembolism in the femoral artery.

Putting It All Together

- It is difficult to link intraoperative events with postoperative CNS injury.
- Many patients have MRI findings of ischemic brain injury—if examined—but few neurologic deficits.
- Endovascular clot retrieval is an option after stroke and could be offered.
- Seizures are often single events, and antiepileptic treatment is rarely needed.
- Brachial plexus lesion may be a cause of postoperative hemiplegia.

> **By the Way**
>
> - Carotid endarterectomy may not prevent postoperative stroke.
> - The value of cerebral monitoring during cardiac surgery is unproven.
> - Preoperative neurologic status is a predictor of postoperative outcome.
> - Postoperative delirium is more common than seizures or stroke.

> **Neurologic Complications After Cardiac Surgery by the Numbers**
>
> - ~40% of patients with postoperative delirium have later cognitive impairment.
> - ~5% of patients develop an ischemic stroke after CABG and valve surgery.
> - ~2% of patients develop ischemic stroke after CABG alone.
> - ~1% of patients develop seizures and half have CT abnormalities.
> - ~0.5% of patients develop mostly transient plexus injury.

References

1. Aronson S, Dyke CM, Levy JH, et al. Does perioperative systolic blood pressure variability predict mortality after cardiac surgery? An exploratory analysis of the ECLIPSE trials. *Anesth Analg* 2011;113:19–30.
2. Arsenault KA, Yusuf AM, Crystal E, et al. Interventions for preventing post-operative atrial fibrillation in patients undergoing heart surgery. *Cochrane Database Syst Rev* 2013; 1:CD003611.
3. Blacker DJ, Flemming KD, Link MJ, Brown RD Jr. The preoperative cerebrovascular consultation: common cerebrovascular questions before general or cardiac surgery. *Mayo Clin Proc* 2004;79:223–229.
4. Charlson ME, Peterson JC, Krieger KH, et al. Improvement of outcomes after coronary artery bypass II: a randomized trial comparing intraoperative high versus customized mean arterial pressure. *J Card Surg* 2007;22:465–472.
5. Ehrlich MP, McCullough JN, Zhang N, et al. Effect of hypothermia on cerebral blood flow and metabolism in the pig. *Ann Thorac Surg* 2002;73:191–197.
6. Ergin MA, Uysal S, Reich DL, et al. Temporary neurological dysfunction after deep hypothermic circulatory arrest: a clinical marker of long-term functional deficit. *Ann Thorac Surg* 1999;67:1887–1890; discussion 1891–1884.
7. Ferrari R, Vidotto G, Muzzolon C, Auriemma S, Salvador L. Neurocognitive deficit and quality of life after mitral valve repair. *J Heart Valve Dis* 2014;23:72–78.
8. Fischer GW, Lin HM, Krol M, et al. Noninvasive cerebral oxygenation may predict outcome in patients undergoing aortic arch surgery. *J Thorac Cardiovasc Surg* 2011;141:815–821.
9. Goldstone AB, Bronster DJ, Anyanwu AC, et al. Predictors and outcomes of seizures after cardiac surgery: a multivariable analysis of 2,578 patients. *Ann Thorac Surg* 2011;91:514–518.
10. Gottesman RF, Sherman PM, Grega MA, et al. Watershed strokes after cardiac surgery: diagnosis, etiology, and outcome. *Stroke* 2006;37:2306–2311.
11. Hedberg M, Boivie P, Engstrom KG. Early and delayed stroke after coronary surgery: an analysis of risk factors and the impact on short- and long-term survival. *Eur J Cardiothorac Surg* 2011;40:379–387.
12. Hui FK, Bain M, Obuchowski NA, et al. Mycotic aneurysm detection rates with cerebral angiography in patients with infective endocarditis. *J Neurointerv Surg* 2015;7:449–452.

13. Hunter GR, Young GB. Seizures after cardiac surgery. *J Cardiothorac Vasc Anesth* 2011; 25:299–305.
14. Lamy A, Devereaux PJ, Prabhakaran D, et al. Effects of off-pump and on-pump coronary-artery bypass grafting at 1 year. *N Engl J Med* 2013;368:1179–1188.
15. Lecker I, Wang DS, Romaschin AD, et al. Tranexamic acid concentrations associated with human seizures inhibit glycine receptors. *J Clin Invest* 2012;122:4654–4666.
16. Mack MJ. Can we make stroke during cardiac surgery a never event? *Thorac Cardiovasc Surg J Thorac Cardiovasc Surg* 2015;149:965–967.
17. Maekawa K, Goto T, Baba T, et al. Abnormalities in the brain before elective cardiac surgery detected by diffusion-weighted magnetic resonance imaging. *Ann Thorac Surg* 2008; 86:1563–1569.
18. Manji RA, Grocott HP, Leake J, et al. Seizures following cardiac surgery: the impact of tranexamic acid and other risk factors. *Can J Anaesth* 2012;59:6–13.
19. Martin K, Knorr J, Breuer T, et al. Seizures after open heart surgery: comparison of epsilon-aminocaproic acid and tranexamic acid. *J Cardiothorac Vasc Anesth* 2011;25:20–25.
20. McCullough JN, Zhang N, Reich DL, et al. Cerebral metabolic suppression during hypothermic circulatory arrest in humans. *Ann Thorac Surg* 1999;67:1895–1899; discussion 1919-1821.
21. McDonagh DL, Berger M, Mathew JP, et al. Neurological complications of cardiac surgery. *Lancet Neurol* 2014;13:490–502.
22. Messé SR, Acker MA, Kasner SE, et al. Determining Neurologic Outcome From Valve Operations (DeNOVO) investigators. Stroke after aortic valve surgery: results from a prospective cohort. *Circulation* 2014;129 2253–2261.
23. Misfeld M, Girrbach F, Etz CD, et al. Surgery for infective endocarditis complicated by cerebral embolism: a consecutive series of 375 patients. *J Thorac Cardiovasc Surg* 2014; 147:1837–1844.
24. Percy A, Widman S, Rizzo JA, Tranquilli M, Elefteriades JA. Deep hypothermic circulatory arrest in patients with high cognitive needs: full preservation of cognitive abilities. *Ann Thorac Surg* 2009;87:117–123.
25. Restrepo L, Wityk RJ, Grega MA, et al. Diffusion- and perfusion-weighted magnetic resonance imaging of the brain before and after coronary artery bypass grafting surgery. *Stroke* 2002;33:2909–2915.
26. Rodriguez RA, Rubens FD, Wozny D, Nathan HJ. Cerebral emboli detected by transcranial Doppler during cardiopulmonary bypass are not correlated with postoperative cognitive deficits. *Stroke* 2010;41:2229–2235.
27. Rossi M, Gallo A, De Silva RJ, Sayeed R. What is the optimal timing for surgery in infective endocarditis with cerebrovascular complications? *Interact Cardiovasc Thorac Surg* 2012;14:72–80.
28. Schlag MG, Hopf R, Redl H. Convulsive seizures following subdural application of fibrin sealant containing tranexamic acid in a rat model. *Neurosurgery* 2000;47:1463–1467.
29. Schmidt R, Enzinger C, Ropele S, Schmidt H, Fazekas F. Progression of cerebral white matter lesions: 6-year results of the Austrian Stroke Prevention Study. *Lancet* 2003; 361:2046–2048.
30. Selnes OA, Gottesman RF, Grega MA, et al. Cognitive and neurologic outcomes after coronary-artery bypass surgery. *N Engl J Med* 2012;366:250–257.
31. Sun X, Lindsay J, Monsein LH, Hill PC, Corso PJ. Silent brain injury after cardiac surgery—a review: cognitive dysfunction and magnetic resonance imaging diffusion-weighted imaging findings. *J Am Coll Cardiol* 2012;60:791–797.
32. Tarakji KG, Sabik JF 3rd, Bhudia SK, Batizy LH, Blackstone EH. Temporal onset, risk factors, and outcomes associated with stroke after coronary artery bypass grafting. *JAMA* 2011;305:381–390.
33. Tully PJ, Baker RA. Current readings: neurocognitive impairment and clinical implications after cardiac surgery. *Semin Thorac Cardiovasc Surg* 2013;25:237–244.

34. Wan S, Sung K, Park PW, et al. Stroke is not a treatment dilemma for early valve surgery in active infective endocarditis. *J Heart Valve Dis* 2014;23:609–616.
35. Whitlock R, Healey JS, Connolly SJ, et al. Predictors of early and late stroke following cardiac surgery. *Can Med Assoc J* 2014;186:905–911.
36. Zheng F, Sheinberg R, Yee MS, et al. Cerebral near-infrared spectroscopy monitoring and neurologic outcomes in adult cardiac surgery patients: a systematic review. *Anesth Analg* 2013;116:663–676.

5

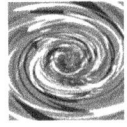

Neurologic Urgencies After Vascular Surgery

Symptomatic vascular disease often leads to vascular surgery. Much of it is elective, but life-threatening emergencies do occur, particularly with rupture of the thoracoabdominal aorta. This may lead to open surgery or endovascular treatment. When neurologic complications occur with aortic surgery, a consultation will usually involve assessment and management of spinal cord ischemia (SCI). The management in most institutions is directed by surgical anesthesiologists, but neurologists may be asked to assess the extent of the damage, which could lead to changes in management. Once threatened, spinal cord tissue may be potentially salvaged by improvement in perfusion, augmentation of blood pressure, and cerebrospinal fluid (CSF) diversion.

One other major vascular procedure is carotid revascularization, which may involve symptomatic or asymptomatic patients. A large proportion of these patients are treated by vascular surgeons. Patients may be in general surgical intensive care units to allow closer postoperative monitoring. Neurologic complications are not common, but they are reasons for urgent consultation.

Many of the major neurologic complications are immediately evident after surgery. In some patients, ischemic stroke becomes apparent in the recovery room. In others, a fatal intracranial hemorrhage caused by a reperfusion syndrome occurs soon after surgery. Lesions of the cranial nerves are of considerable postoperative concern—difficulty with swallowing and coughing may be the first sign. The main questions a consulting neurologist will have to ask are the following: Is there evidence of a complete or incomplete SCI? Is the patient adequately managed with blood pressure augmentation and CSF drainage? Does the patient have an ischemic stroke after carotid surgery, and if so, why? Is an endovascular procedure indicated? This chapter provides guidance when consulting on these (largely unexpected) complications after major vascular procedures.

Principles

When discussing strategies to reduce or mitigate neurologic complications, some background information is needed. Two major vascular surgeries are discussed here. Each has specific problems to consider.

BLOOD SUPPLY TO SPINAL CORD

It is important to appreciate the highly variable vascular anatomy of the spine and how it may lead to complications. This knowledge can then be used to understand the risks to perfusion of the cord. First, the aorta provides multiple intercostal arteries and lumbar arteries, which split into anterior and posterior radicular arteries and then into the anterior and posterior spinal arteries. The anterior spinal artery enters the cord through a sulcal artery. This sulcal artery typically provides blood to the lateral corticospinal tracts (motor function) and is placed medially. The more anterior lateral spinothalamic tract (sensory function) does receive blood not from the sulcal artery but from branches coming off the anterior spinal artery (the coronary arteries). This may explain the discrepancy between a full anterior spinal syndrome and a more central cord syndrome in which the coronary arteries are preserved, resulting in a centrally located infarction.

Again, the intercostal arteries are the main source of blood to the cord; this is why they are predictably compromised with aortic dissection, which rips them piece by piece. These intercostal arteries that branch out to radicular arteries have many individual variations. There is a cervicothoracic area (cervical cord and thoracic segments T1 and T2) where these radicular arteries branch out from the vertebral artery and costocervical trunk. Thus, vertebral artery injury may cause ischemic cervical cord syndromes. There is a thoracolumbar area starting from T3 with a large radicular artery (the arteria radicularis magna, or artery of Adamkiewicz). This artery is crucial to perfusion of the thoracic spinal cord, but its location (to be identified by vascular surgeons) varies between T2 and L2 (usually between T9 and T12). The sacral areas of the cord (cauda equina) are perfused by a different set of arteries, namely branches of the internal iliac and middle sacral artery (Figure 5.1). Therefore, the midthoracic region is the most vulnerable area, but lesions are often located at the level of T4 (nipple) or T10 (navel). The venous system consists of single anterior and posterior veins that drain into the paravertebral plexus and the venous systems of the pelvis.

The physics of blood and CSF circulation in the spinal cord are the same as in the brain. Cerebrospinal pressure is the arterial pressure minus the venous pressure. Increased venous pressure may lead to increased spinal CSF pressure with reduced spinal artery flow and reduced spinal cord perfusion. The system is also autoregulated within a certain range of blood pressures (Figure 5.2).[17] There is little information as to how anesthetic agents change spinal cord flow autoregulation and what early ischemia does to these curves (i.e., increase or decrease spinal cord flow). Interestingly, there is evidence of a positive effect of ischemic preconditioning.[25]

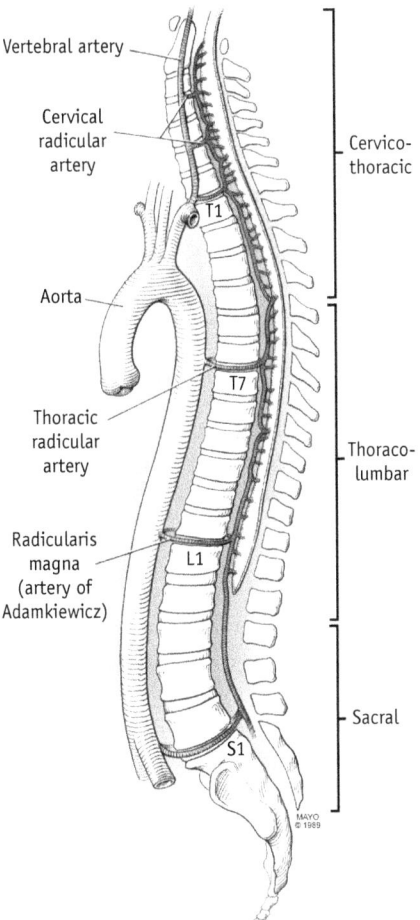

Figure 5.1 Vascularization of the spinal cord, showing cervical (C), thoracic (T), and lumbar (L) regions. From Wijdicks.[46]

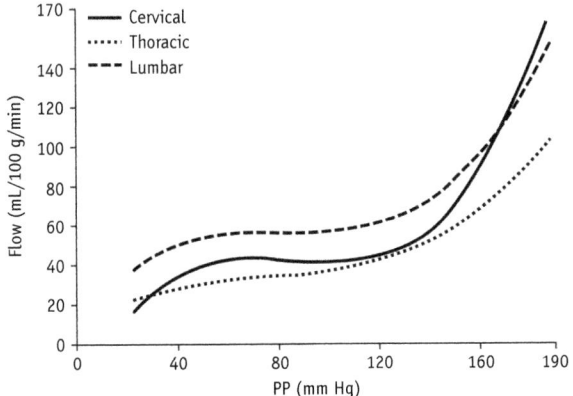

Figure 5.2 Autoregulatory curves for cervical, thoracic, and lumbar spinal cord blood flow in response to changes in perfusion pressure (PP). Adapted from Hickey et al.[17]

Increasing the "resilience" of the spinal cord has found its way into elective management of aortic aneurysm with a combination of endovascular (first stage) and open surgery.[13]

In order to understand how aneurysm localization may impair spinal cord flow, it is important to have a good understanding of the Crawford classification of thoracoabdominal aneurysms:

- Type I is a thoracic aneurysm that extends inferiorly to the extent that it involves the visceral vessels.
- Type II is a diffuse thoracoabdominal aneurysm with extensive involvement of the aorta both above and below the visceral arteries.
- Type III has aneurysmal changes that begin below the middle of the thoracic aorta.
- Type IV consists of aneurysmal changes that start at the level of the diaphragm and involve both the visceral vessels and the infrarenal aorta.

The risk of cord ischemia is related to the type of thoracoabdominal aneurysm repair (Figure 5.3).

The spinal cord is immediately compromised after aortic declamping; this paradox is explained by the profound hypotension that results from reperfusion of ischemic vasodilated and vasomotor paralyzed lower extremities. Anesthesiologists are well tuned into this critical phase of surgery and usually use volume loading preemptively and boluses of vasopressors. In addition, the concentration of ventilation agents is reduced before clamp relief.

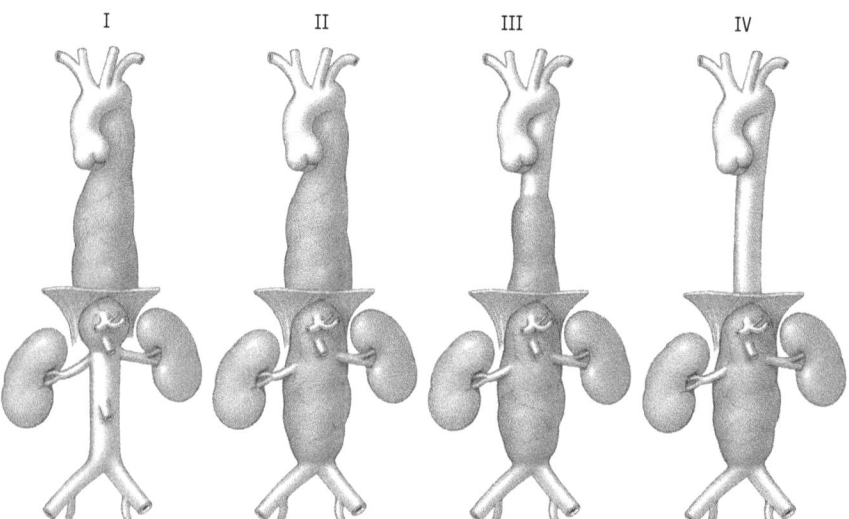

Figure 5.3 Maximal reported incidences of paraplegia by Crawford's classification: Surgical repair type I, 7%; type II, 24%; type III, 22%; type IV, 13%; Endovascular repair type I, 10%; type II, 10%; type III, 19%; type IV, 5%; From Wijdicks.[45]

Usually, prolonged clamping increases the risk of postoperative SCI. The risk increases significantly after 30 minutes of clamping and doubles with any additional 30 minutes of clamping. More than 60 minutes of cross-clamp time has in some studies been associated with 24% risk of paraplegia. Many cardiothoracic surgeons routinely reimplant the intercostal arteries, but others question whether the incidence of paraplegia can be reduced by such a time-consuming procedure. The cardiothoracic surgeon therefore is faced with the dilemma of reimplanting as many intercostal arteries as possible (requiring an estimated 10 minutes for end-to-end anastomosis), with the assumption that one or more critical intercostal arteries will be included, or proceeding directly to replace the aneurysm within a short clamping time.

The main pathophysiology of spinal cord injury has simply to do with altered blood flow mechanics that are associated with aortic cross-clamping. Most of the time, the watershed area in the midthoracic (T4 to T8) level is most at risk. This area may also be compromised if there are a reduced number of radicular arteries. Some have argued that there is a reperfusion phase that may be damaging, but trials of postreperfusion hypothermia have not led to a significant change in the incidence of paraplegia.

OPERATIVE MANAGEMENT OF AORTIC DISEASE

Intraoperative protection of the spinal cord has evolved from reducing aortic clamp time and "racing against the clock" to reimplant as many segmental arteries as possible to use of atrial-femoral bypass circuits with one cannula into the left atrium and one in the femoral artery, providing retrograde blood supply to the spinal cord.[9,12] This procedure is often used in combination with CSF drainage, and the reduction in spinal cord injury has been dramatic in more risky cases (from almost 10% to 1–2%).

Surgery can be divided into elective and emergent repair. With elective surgery, the perioperative management of an aortic repair can begin before the patient enters the operating room. The goals of blood pressure control during a presenting dissection are much less clearly defined, with some experts accepting systolic pressures in the range of 100 mm Hg as long as patient alertness is not compromised. Reducing aortic wall stress may be arbitrarily achieved by keeping the heart rate slower than 60 beats per minute and the systolic blood pressure at least less than 120 mm Hg. Fluids should be used cautiously because they may dilute coagulation factors and disrupt thrombi.[9,18,29]

As alluded to earlier, the most challenging part for the anesthesiologist is the aortic cross-clamping and unclamping.[14] This involves discontinuation of venodilators, vasopressors, and fluids and general avoidance of arteriolar dilators that can affect distal aortic pressure. Hypotension in the postoperative phase may be caused by a retroperitoneal hematoma or by ischemic adrenal insufficiency, both of which require acute intervention.[3] During surgery, normothermia is maintained, and outcome may be related to intraoperative temperatures.[35]

Emergent intervention is obviously quite different, and many factors play a crucial role. This includes selection of patients by the surgeon. Emergency repair is mostly for a type A (ascending aorta) dissection. Patients may have an ischemic stroke or SCI at onset. Several patterns have been reported with paraplegia. Mostly, it is a flaccid paraplegia with loss of sensation, but Brown-Sequard syndrome or an acute cauda equina syndrome may occur. These symptoms are often permanent, but there have been reported improvements after repair. Dissection of the descending aorta can cause iliac artery occlusions and ischemic neuropathy, mostly as a result of a (rare) compartment syndrome. Dissection of the descending aorta is a life-threatening condition, and survival may be close to a flip of a coin. Not only do survivors have a much higher risk of spinal cord injury, but also the involvement of the renal arteries can cause acute renal failure requiring dialysis and the involvement of the celiac and mesenteric arteries results in acute necrotic colon and sepsis after resection.

Endovascular management of acute and chronic vascular diseases using a variety of endografts has been attempted in patients with significant medical comorbidity; a lower rate of perioperative paraplegia (2%) has been claimed with this approach compared with prior surgical studies, but the incidence was 13% in one experience mostly with extensive repairs and not related to acuteness of the intervention.[10,40] Factors that increase postoperative paraplegia in endovascular management include infrarenal aorta replacement, extensive stenting of the thoracic aorta, and a compromised hypogastric artery.

OPERATIVE MANAGEMENT OF CAROTID DISEASE

Carotid revascularization remains a very common procedure, but the risk of a complication is not so high.[5,11,34] The reported incidences in clinical trials in no way represent an accurate picture of the true risk. (Come to think of it, if 3 complications occur in 1 month, the surgeon has to show 97 uncomplicated procedures the rest of the year to quote a 3% postoperative risk.) The carotid artery is superficially located in the neck and easily approachable. The arteriotomy is made on the anterior surface of the internal carotid artery. The proximity of the cranial nerves predisposes them to injury during carotid exposure. A recent analysis in 1,151 patients found 4.6% of patients with cranial nerve deficits and with 80% resolution in 1 year.[16] Carotid endarterectomy requires a cross-clamping time of about 30 minutes. The common carotid artery is occluded with a vascular clamp, and smaller clamps or aneurysm clips are used to occlude the internal and external carotid arteries.

Intraoperative shunting is not a universal practice. Some surgeons use a shunt if changes are apparent during electroencephalographic monitoring. In a few patients, shunt placement is technically not possible because of a high bifurcation, distal plaque, or a diminutive internal carotid artery. After removal of gross plaque, a smooth arteriotomy bed is the best result. One of the most important parts of the surgical procedure is to reduce stray adventitial tacks or suture ends sewn into the lumen, because they may eventually produce thrombosis or dissection.

The Carotid Revascularization Endarterectomy Versus Stenting Trial (CREST) found no differences between the two procedures in combining stroke, myocardial infarction, or mortality even when stenting was done with credentialed interventionalists.[6] The risk of stroke in patients older than 70 years of age was increased. The risk of complications with stenting pertains to vessel tortuosity and atherosclerotic buildup in the aortic arch, which may cause embolization even when "protection devices" are navigated through these segments. Restenosis after carotid stenting is low; a 2003 study reported restenosis of 70% or greater in fewer than 2% of patients after a 2-year follow-up period.[7] In a more recent study from the CREST investigators, restenosis and occlusion were higher, approximately 6% for both endarterectomy and stenting.[24]

Cerebral hyperperfusion syndrome, which is highly uncommon (1%), is seen with equal frequency in both carotid endarterectomies and carotid artery stenting syndromes.[26] The current view is that cerebral autoregulation is impaired in patients who have severe carotid artery stenosis and that those with more severe stenosis have more severe impairments. After endarterectomy, the increase in pressure in capillaries and vessels that are maximally dilated causes disruption of epithelial cells and breakdown of the blood–brain barrier. This effect is most pronounced during the first week after carotid endarterectomy. Although systemic hypertension is the primary event leading to intracranial hemorrhage after carotid endarterectomy, anticoagulation may also contribute to the development of a hemorrhage. Patients develop severe unilateral headache and a new hemiparesis, and a new hemorrhage is seen in the anterior cerebral circulation.

In Practice

It remains surprising that the incidence of paraplegia after major vascular repairs—at least in large, experienced centers—is approximately 4%. There is some variability, with some centers reporting significantly higher rates (10%–20%), but this can be explained by the heterogeneity (with more extensive repairs and major comorbidity) of most reported surgical series. Even with this low incidence, the handicap is devastating and measures should be in place to prevent ischemia of the spinal cord.[20,39,44] Spinal cord injury after elective or emergent repair is usually present immediately; more rarely, it may emerge later.[30]

Spinal cord injury after aortic dissection is another vascular catastrophe, but whether paraplegia occurs is not related to the extent of intercostal artery involvement in the field of the dissection. A much more likely mechanism is hypoperfusion of the spinal cord associated with profound shock. Cardiogenic shock from aortic dissection is caused by severe aortic regurgitation and cardiac tamponade with hemopericardium. Syncope is relatively common in aortic dissection and may be related

Table 5.1 **Management of Acute Spinal Cord Ischemia**

- CSF (lumbar) drainage for 24–48 hours
- Aim at a CSF pressure of 8–12 mm Hg
- Increase MAP by 10 mm Hg every 5 minutes until improvement or when MAP of 130 mm Hg is reached
- MRI of the spine for epidural hematoma or assessment of ischemia
- Monitor neurologic exam frequently
- Maintain MAP for 1–2 days and gradually wean

CSF, cerebrospinal fluid; MAP, mean arterial pressure; MRI, magnetic resonance imaging. Adapted from reference 20.

to acute hypotension caused by cardiac tamponade or aortic rupture, cerebral vessel obstruction, or damage to the carotid baroreceptors. The outcome of paraplegia in dissection of the aorta is similarly poor.

The initial assessment should involve determination of a complete or incomplete spinal cord infarction. Involvement of the corticospinal, pyramidal, and spinothalamic tracts and anterior horns results in flaccid paraplegia. Pinprick and hot and cold sensation are absent, but light touch and position sense are spared, and there is a reduced sensation to the level of the nipples at T4. Loss of rectal sphincter tone is common. Paraplegia of the flaccid type may occur, but there also may be paraplegia in extension or flexion, particularly in partial lesions. Flexor reflex may occur later as a manifestation of (often violent) spasms, or earlier when the spinal shock phase passes. The bladder is dysfunctional and retention occurs, potentially leading to renal failure with rising creatinine levels and is prevented by immediate catheterization.

Although there is no proof of efficacy and just a few physicians are convinced, many patients with a spinal cord injury will be treated with lumbar spinal CSF drainage.[2,19,22,23,48] This reduces the intraspinal pressure and may improve perfusion. Most of the time, the goal of CSF drainage is to maintain a spinal pressure of less than 10 mm Hg (Table 5.1). Many institutions recommend a maximal drainage rate of 20 mL/h (about the same as hourly production of CSF). This is continued for 24–48 hours, and then the drain is clamped—if the patient is asymptomatic or unchanged, the lumbar drain is removed. Very few complications are seen with CSF drainage through a well placed drain. Catheter-related morbidity is low, on the order of 4%, and in a large study of 135 treated patients, no spinal epidural hematomas were found.[48] Delayed spinal cord injury is rare and more likely represents a delayed discovery, although convincing cases of patients with an asymptomatic postoperative interval have been published. Systemic hypotension has frequently been implicated, because some patients improve after the blood pressure is improved. Some have treated these patients with an additional high dose of methylprednisolone (1,000 mg IV).[1,4,15,37]

Urgent consultation for a possible complication of carotid surgery may involve assessment for possible ischemic stroke or management of blood pressure and heart

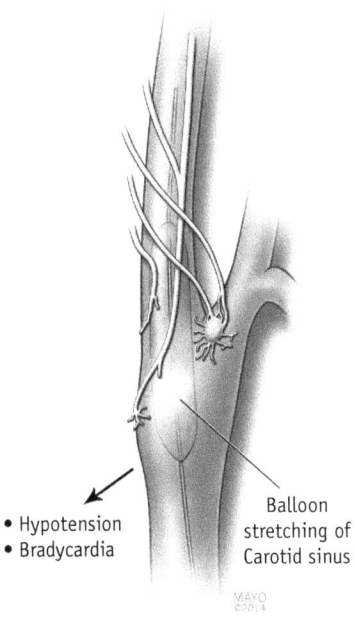

Figure 5.4 Stenting of the carotid artery and relation to baroreceptors.

rate instability. The latter condition is mostly managed by a neurointensivist, but a general neurologist should be aware of this major complication involving damage to the baroreceptors.

Carotid stenting can cause significant baroreceptor dysfunction due to balloon stretching of the vessel before actual stent placement (Figure 5-4).[41–43] Postoperative hypotension may last 48 hours or even up to 1 week.[47] It is often associated with bradycardia. Phenylephrine administered through a central access catheter may be needed, with attempts at weaning 24 hours later. Midodrine (up to 15 mg four times daily) may be a good transitional drug. Risk factors for hypotension include multiple dilatations, balloon angioplasty to greater than 8 atm, and prior use of β-blockage. Fluid bolus may be needed, along with intravenous atropine (0.5-mg increments).[28,32] Because many patients have coexisting congestive heart failure, fluid bolus should be used sparingly and it is much safer to provide support with vasopressors in this category of patients. A predictive scoring system has been developed (Table 5.2). A score of 4 predicts prolonged hypotension, and a score of 2 predicts transient hypotension.

Commonly, carotid artery endarterectomy is without any postoperative complications. Rare complications include carotid hematoma resulting in acute carotid

Table 5.2 **Prediction of Hypotension After Carotid Artery Stenting**

Findings	Risk Factor
Distance from carotid bifurcation to maximum stenotic lesion	
<10 mm	1
>10 mm	0
Type of stenosis	
Eccentric	1
Concentric	0
Plaque morphology	
Echogenic	1
Intermediate~echolucent	0
Calcification at carotid bifurcation	
Calcification (+)	1
Calcification (−)	0
Total	**4**

From Nonaka et al.[32]

occlusion and new neurologic signs and thromboembolic events during the procedure.

Perioperative strokes after revascularization of the carotid artery are usually found immediately after presentation.[21,27] Most postoperative strokes result from thrombosis or a dissection of the operated segment that causes partial or complete occlusion. Wall hematoma (carotid blowout) is rare and is often recognized by a rapidly growing neck mass. Extravasation leads to suffocation, and emergency intubation is needed even if the neck mass is still small. Because the trachea can rapidly become compressed, it is ill advised to wait to obtain studies (i.e., computed tomography angiography) before securing the airway. With documented carotid occlusions, some surgeons have decided to reoperate in the same field and try to re-open the artery. In one large trial (North American Symptomatic Carotid Endarterectomy Trial, 5 of 13 patients had reoperation for carotid occlusion and improved, but in general, only half of reoperated patients achieve a good functional outcome.[36,38,45,49]

Acute carotid stent thrombosis is a rare complication, reportedly occurring in up to 2% of patients, and has been attributed to failure to treat with dual antiplatelet therapy. These patients can benefit from the administration of glycoprotein IIb/IIIa receptor antagonists such as IV abciximab or tirofiban. Endovascular management may also be considered, but there are very few data demonstrating improved outcome.

In many patients, improvements in hemodynamic stabilization and augmentation might decrease the size of the infarction.

Cerebral hyperperfusion syndrome is difficult to manage. Some surgeons have, in desperation, evacuated the hematoma, but with substantial postoperative morbidity and often de-escalation of care if the patient is injured to a great extent. Tight control of blood pressure may be the only option—next to the usual β-blockade (IV labetalol), calcium channel blockers (IV nicardipine) or clonidine because it is a potent sympatholytic and decreases heart rate, blood pressure, and cardiac output. If there is substantial cerebral edema surrounding the hematoma, mannitol or hypertonic saline in scheduled doses is needed. Cerebral hyperperfusion syndrome with intracranial hematoma is devastating. Cerebral hyperperfusion without hematoma—persistent headache and hemiparesis with brain edema alone—has a much better outcome with much lower mortality and even morbidity—most patients recover fully.[34]

A recent review from the United Kingdom suggested that three strategies can reduce complications after carotid endarterectomy:[31] (1) use of transcranial Doppler ultrasound (detection of emboli in middle cerebral artery) or angioscopy (direct visualization) to detect retained luminal thrombus before flow restoration, (2) institution of dual antiplatelet therapy to prevent postoperative thrombus formation and possibly perioperative cardiac events, and (3) institution of a clear protocol for treating hypertension after cardiac endarterectomy (defined as systolic blood pressure >160 mm Hg), escalating from labetalol infusion of 50 mg/h to 10 mg hydralazine IV.

Putting It All Together

- There are limited options for treatment of immediate paraplegia.
- There is potential for benefit with CSF drainage in the delayed-onset type of paraplegia.
- Ischemic stroke after carotid endarterectomy or stenting is uncommon, but may require acute endovascular intervention.
- Baroreceptor damage from angioplasty can result in several days of hypotension and bradycardia.
- Cerebral hyperperfusion syndrome is most common in patients with a very tight carotid artery stenosis.
- Cerebral hyperperfusion syndrome requires acute medical and surgical intervention in patients who have a large cerebral hematoma and surrounding edema.

> **By the Way**
>
> - Complications of lumbar drain placement include infection from ongoing leakage around the insertion site.
> - Acute postoperative carotid artery occlusion requires decompressive hemicraniectomy in a large proportion of patients.
> - Preoperative evaluation of hyperperfusion by single-photon emission computed tomography with acetazolamide can be performed and identifies patients at risk, but may not prevent occurrence.

> **Neurologic Complications of Vascular Surgery by the Numbers**
>
> - ~10% of patients have a postoperative stroke after urgent repair of TAA
> - ~5% of patients with carotid stenting develop hypotension and bradycardia.
> - ~5% of patients may have SCI after TAA rupture and open repair.
> - ~4% of patients may have SCI after TAA rupture and TEVAR.[40]
> - ~4% of patients may have stroke after TAA rupture and TEVAR.
> - ~1% of patients develop cerebral hyperperfusion syndrome.

References

1. Bajwa A, Davis M, Moawad M, Taylor PR. Paraplegia following elective endovascular repair of abdominal aortic aneurysm: reversal with cerebrospinal fluid drainage. *Eur J Vasc Endovasc Surg* 2008;35:46–48.
2. Bilal H, O'Neill B, Mahmood S, Waterworth P. Is cerebrospinal fluid drainage of benefit to neuroprotection in patients undergoing surgery on the descending thoracic aorta or thoracoabdominal aorta? *Interact Cardiovasc Thorac Surg* 2012;15:702–708.
3. Bjorck M, Wanhainen A, Djavani K, Acosta S. The clinical importance of monitoring intra-abdominal pressure after ruptured abdominal aortic aneurysm repair. *Scand J Surg* 2008;97:183–190.
4. Blacker DJ, Wijdicks EF, Ramakrishna G. Resolution of severe paraplegia due to aortic dissection after CSF drainage. *Neurology* 2003;61:142–143.
5. Bradac O, Mohapl M, Kramar F, et al. Carotid endarterectomy and carotid artery stenting: changing paradigm during 10 years in a high-volume centre. *Acta Neurochir (Wien)* 2014;156:1705–1712.
6. Brott TG, Hobson RW 2nd, Howard G, et al. Stenting versus endarterectomy for treatment of carotid-artery stenosis. *N Engl J Med* 2010;363:11–23.
7. Cernetti C, Reimers B, Picciolo A, et al. Carotid artery stenting with cerebral protection in 100 consecutive patients: immediate and two-year follow-up results. *Ital Heart J* 2003;4:695–700.
8. Chaikof EL, Brewster DC, Dalman RL, et al. The care of patients with an abdominal aortic aneurysm: the Society for Vascular Surgery practice guidelines. *J Vasc Surg* 2009;50:S2–S49.

9. Conrad MF, Ergul EA, Patel VI, et al. Evolution of operative strategies in open thoracoabdominal aneurysm repair. *J Vasc Surg* 2011;53:1195–1201.e1.
10. Dias NV, Sonesson B, Kristmundsson T, et al. Short-term outcome of spinal cord ischemia after endovascular repair of thoracoabdominal aortic aneurysms. *Eur J Vasc Endovasc Surg.* 2015;49:403–409.
11. Eller JL, Snyder KV, Siddiqui AH, Levy EI, Hopkins LN. Endovascular treatment of carotid stenosis. *Neurosurg Clin North Am* 2014;25:565–582.
12. Estrera AL, Miller CC 3rd, Chen EP, et al. Descending thoracic aortic aneurysm repair: 12-year experience using distal aortic perfusion and cerebrospinal fluid drainage. *Ann Thorac Surg* 2005;80:1290–1296.
13. Etz DC, Luehr M, Aspern KV, et al. Spinal cord ischemia in open and endovascular thoracoabdominal aortic aneurysm repair: new concepts. *J Cardiovasc Surg* 2014;55:159–168.
14. Gelman S. The pathophysiology of aortic cross-clamping and unclamping. *Anesthesiology* 1995;82:1026–1060.
15. Goldstein LJ, Rezayat C, Shrikhande GV, Bush HL Jr. Delayed permanent paraplegia after endovascular repair of abdominal aortic aneurysm. *J Vasc Surg* 2010;51:725–728.
16. Hye RJ, Mackey A, Hill MD, et al. Incidence, outcomes, and effect on quality of life of cranial nerve injury in the Carotid Revascularization Endarterectomy versus Stenting Trial. *J Vasc Surg* 2015;61:1208–1215.
17. Hickey R, Albin MS, Bunegin L, Gelineau J. Autoregulation of spinal cord blood flow: is the cord a microcosm of the brain? *Stroke* 1986;17:1183–1189.
18. Hiratzka LF, Bakris GL, Beckman JA, et al. 2010 ACCF/AHA/AATS/ACR/ASA/SCA/SCAI/SIR/STS/SVM guidelines for the diagnosis and management of patients with thoracic aortic disease: a report of the American College of Cardiology Foundation/American Heart Association Task Force on Practice Guidelines, American Association for Thoracic Surgery, American College of Radiology, American Stroke Association, Society of Cardiovascular Anesthesiologists, Society for Cardiovascular Angiography and Interventions, Society of Interventional Radiology, Society of Thoracic Surgeons, and Society for Vascular Medicine. *Circulation* 2010;121:e266–e369.
19. Hnath JC, Mehta M, Taggert JB, et al. Strategies to improve spinal cord ischemia in endovascular thoracic aortic repair: outcomes of a prospective cerebrospinal fluid drainage protocol. *J Vasc Surg* 2008;48:836–840.
20. Hogendoorn W, Schlosser FJ, Muhs BE, Popescu WM. Surgical and anesthetic considerations for the endovascular treatment of ruptured descending thoracic aortic aneurysms. *Curr Opin Anaesthesiol* 2014;27:12–20.
21. Jacobowitz GR, Rockman CB, Lamparello PJ, et al. Causes of perioperative stroke after carotid endarterectomy: special considerations in symptomatic patients. *Ann Vasc Surg* 2001;15:19–24.
22. Keith CJ Jr, Passman MA, Carignan MJ, et al. Protocol implementation of selective postoperative lumbar spinal drainage after thoracic aortic endograft. *J Vasc Surg* 2012;55:1–8; discussion 8.
23. Khan SN, Stansby G. Cerebrospinal fluid drainage for thoracic and thoracoabdominal aortic aneurysm surgery. *Cochrane Database Syst Rev* 2012;10:CD003635.
24. Lal BK, Beach KW, Roubin GS, et al. Restenosis after carotid artery stenting and endarterectomy: a secondary analysis of CREST, a randomized controlled trial. *Lancet Neurol* 2012;11:755–763.
25. Liang CL, Lu K, Liliang PC, et al. Ischemic preconditioning ameliorates spinal cord ischemia-reperfusion injury by triggering autoregulation. *J Vasc Surg* 2012;55:1116–1123.
26. Lieb M, Shah U, Hines GL. Cerebral hyperperfusion syndrome after carotid intervention: a review. *Cardiol Rev* 2012;20:84–89.
27. Macdonald S. Carotid artery stenting trials: conduct, results, critique, and current recommendations. *Cardiovasc Intervent Radiol* 2012;35:15–29.

28. Mlekusch W, Schillinger M, Sabeti S, et al. Hypotension and bradycardia after elective carotid stenting: frequency and risk factors. *J Endovasc Ther* 2003;10:851–859
29. Moll FL, Powell JT, Fraedrich G, et al. Management of abdominal aortic aneurysms: clinical practice guidelines of the European society for vascular surgery. *Eur J Vasc Endovasc Surg* 2011;41 Suppl 1:S1–S58.
30. Nasr B, Schneider F, Marques da Fonseca P, Gouny P. Cholesterol crystal embolism and delayed-onset paraplegia after thoracoabdominal aneurysm repair. *Ann Vasc Surg* 2014;28:1320 e1321–e1323.
31. Naylor AR, Sayers RD, McCarthy MJ, et al. Closing the loop: a 21-year audit of strategies for preventing stroke and death following carotid endarterectomy. *Eur J Vasc Endovasc Surg* 2013;46:161–170.
32. Nonaka T, Oka S, Miyata K, et al. Prediction of prolonged postprocedural hypotension after carotid artery stenting. *Neurosurgery* 2005;57:472–477.
33. O'Brien M, Chandra A. Carotid revascularization: risks and benefits. *Vasc Health Risk Manag* 2014;10:403–416.
34. Ogasawara K, Mikami C, Inoue T, Ogawa A. Delayed cerebral hyperperfusion syndrome caused by prolonged impairment of cerebrovascular autoregulation after carotid endarterectomy: case report. *Neurosurgery* 2004;54:1258–1261.
35. Quiroga E, Tran NT, Hatsukami T, Starnes BW. Hypothermia is associated with increased mortality in patients undergoing repair of ruptured abdominal aortic aneurysm. *J Endovasc Ther* 2010;17:434–438.
36. Radak D, Popovic AD, Radicevic S, Neskovic AN, Bojic M. Immediate reoperation for perioperative stroke after 2250 carotid endarterectomies: differences between intraoperative and early postoperative stroke. *J Vasc Surg* 1999;30:245–251.
37. Riess KP, Gundersen SB 3rd, Ziegelbein KJ. Delayed neurologic deficit after infrarenal endovascular aortic aneurysm repair. *Am Surg* 2007;73:385–387.
38. Rockman CB, Jacobowitz GR, Lamparello PJ, et al. Immediate reexploration for the perioperative neurologic event after carotid endarterectomy: is it worthwhile? *J Vasc Surg* 2000;32:1062–1070.
39. Sadek M, Abjigitova D, Pellet Y, et al. Operative outcomes after open repair of descending thoracic aortic aneurysms in the era of endovascular surgery. *Ann Thorac Surg* 2014;97:1562–1567.
40. Schlosser FJ, Verhagen HJ, Lin PH, et al. TEVAR following prior abdominal aortic aneurysm surgery: increased risk of neurological deficit. *J Vasc Surg* 2009;49:308–314; discussion 314.
41. Tarlov E, Schmidek H, Scott RM, Wepsic JG, Ojemann RG. Reflex hypotension following carotid endarterectomy: mechanism and management. *J Neurosurg* 1973;39:323–327.
42. Tyden G, Samnegard H, Thulin L. Rational treatment of hypotension after carotid endarterectomy by carotid sinus nerve blockade. *Acta Chir Scand Suppl* 1980;500:61–64.
43. Tyden G, Samnegard H, Thulin L, Muhrbeck O. Effect of carotid endarterectomy on baroreflex sensitivity in man: intraoperative studies. *Acta Chir Scand Suppl* 1980;500:67–69.
44. Ullery BW, Cheung AT, Fairman RM, et al. Risk factors, outcomes, and clinical manifestations of spinal cord ischemia following thoracic endovascular aortic repair. *J Vasc Surg* 2011;54:677–684.
45. Van den Berg JC. Neuro-rescue during carotid stenting. *Eur J Vasc Endovasc Surg* 2008;36:627–636.
46. Wijdicks EFM. *Neurologic Complications of Critical Illness*. 3rd ed. Oxford: Oxford University Press, 2009.
47. Winters HS, Anderson C, Parker G. Prolonged hypotension following elective stenting of an internal carotid artery stenosis. *J Neurointerv Surg* 2014;7:e4.

48. Wong CS, Healy D, Canning C, et al. A systematic review of spinal cord injury and cerebrospinal fluid drainage after thoracic aortic endografting. *J Vasc Surg* 2012;56:1438–1447.
49. Wu TY, Anderson NE, Barber PA. Neurological complications of carotid revascularisation. *J Neurol Neurosurg Psychiatry* 2012;83:543–550.

6

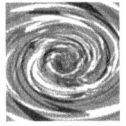

Post–Cardiac Arrest Support and the Brain

A frequent reason for a neurology consult in the intensive care unit (ICU) is to assess a comatose patient after cardiopulmonary resuscitation (CPR) and adequate resumption of spontaneous circulation. This is also one of the most difficult tasks. Cynics may argue that the neurologist may not be needed to assess the prognosis of a comatose patient one or two days after CPR—the patient's chances for good recovery are poor. Unfortunately there is a misconception that is all there is to it. The rate of mortality and poor outcome in most recent studies of surviving comatose patients after CPR however has remained at about 50%.[41,42] The key to successful outcome is having a bystander who not only is able to do CPR but also has knowledge and skill in doing so. Once patients are resuscitated, it is common practice to move them to the coronary artery catheterization suite, and patients may benefit from urgent revascularization.

For the neurologist seeing a patient for the first time, five main questions (as well as subsidiary questions) should be asked: (1) Is there any possibility that cardiac arrest was a consequence of an acute catastrophic intracranial hemorrhage, and what did the computed tomography (CT) scan of the brain show? (2) What is the patient's cardiac reserve, and how advanced is current support? (3) When was hypothermia started, and what supportive medication and in what dose is being used? (4) Is there evidence of liver or kidney injury that could slow drug metabolism? (5) Is electroencephalography (EEG) monitoring in place and warranted, or has a spot EEG excluded ongoing seizures?

Over the last decade, the practice of neurologic assessment of patients with acute severe brain injury after cardiac standstill has become more complicated as a result of cooling, the use of additional sedation and neuromuscular junction blockers, and especially the introduction of extracorporeal membrane oxygenation (ECMO).[27,28,32] With all that noise and confounding, the hands of the neurologist may be tied, and they may just have to deliberatively wait.

This chapter provides three pieces of crucial information. First, current practices of targeted temperature management are reviewed. The term *therapeutic hypothermia*—assuredly called "therapeutic" by strong proponents of the intervention—has commonly been used to set this procedure apart from accidental hypothermia or hypothermia associated with medical or neurologic disease. Now a new term *Targeted Temperature Management* seems to take hold. Cooling of unresponsive resuscitated patients has been considered the standard of care for patients with cardiac arrest due to a shockable rhythm.[45-47,61] Cooling of patients has also been recommended by specifically created councils and guideline committees of US and European professional organizations.[12] Hypothermia with various temperatures is likely effective through abating oxidative stress and reducing excitotoxicity, but six patients must be treated to find benefit for one, reducing its overall effectiveness.[62] Protocols may change in favor of targeted temperature management, aiming at fever control or far more moderate hypothermia at 36°C. Second, this chapter concentrates on the more severely affected patient, one who has required extracorporeal support. Third, the tools of prognostication in comatose patients after CPR are reiterated here, but a more detailed discussion can be found in another volume of this series (*Communicating Prognosis*).

Often, the pendulum has shifted toward the more severely injured patient, who has a much lower probability of a good outcome, but one may still need to identify patients who have a fighting chance. For many intensivists, neurologists seem to be the harbingers of doom (and often they are), but one of the important tasks is to make sure patients are given a fair chance and that withdrawal does not occur as a result of too-quick decision making or faulty perception.

Predictors of poor neurologic outcome (with and without hypothermia) have been systematically reviewed. The guidelines recommended in 2006 by the American Academy of Neurology[63] (discussed in greater detail later) remain valid after additional review of studies, emphasizing the reliability of myoclonus status epilepticus, fixed pupils, and bilateral absence of N20 cortical responses on somatosensory evoked potentials (SSEP) for poor prognosis in most instances. The criterion of low EEG voltage (unreactive and suppressed EEG) has been added, but it is unknown whether it is an independent variable, and, as expected, it is more often seen in patients with the absence of several brainstem reflexes.[53] After therapeutic hypothermia (33°C), one study found that only N20 cortical absence on SSEP, a nonreactive EEG after rewarming, absent oculocephalic responses, and extensor motor responses or worse were predictors with sufficient reliability.[54]

To the reader it will become rapidly clear that studies on prognosis vary because patients vary and the neurologic acumen of the assessing specialist may vary. The assessment and management of comatose patients after return of spontaneous circulation is a major clinical and neurologic task that requires several physicians thinking through the clinical presentation and thus a multidisciplinary approach.

Principles

The first core principle is to have an understanding of the limits of CPR. Cardiac arrest is the most profound injury to the brain, even worse than traumatic brain injury or central nervous system infection. If there is no global arterial supply to neurons, the brain oxygen tension in brain tissue will decline in just a few minutes.[3] This leads to dysfunction of cell membrane ion pumps and then to a rapid unraveling of the cellular machinery, resulting in opening of calcium channels and release of excitatory amino acids eventually, calcium overload and cellular death occurs. This sequence is well established, but what is also well established is that restoration of circulation does not automatically lead to reperfusion. There are many areas that are not reperfused (the *no-flow phenomenon*) as a result of endothelial edema due to ischemia, blood sludging, early intervascular coagulation, and leukocyte adhesion (Figure 6.1).[7,14,34,36] In fact it may be more complex and because of the potent vasoparalysis, a period of hyperperfusion followed by hypoperfusion may occur, resulting in a marked reduction of cerebral blood flow.[24]

The cytopathology of ischemia is impressive with nuclear hyperchromasia, nuclear pyknosis, cytoplasmic eosinophilia, cytoplasmic shrinkage, cytoplasmic microvacuolation, and cell homogenization, and finally total disintegration usually in specific locations such as the hippocampus, thalamus, and cortex.[26]

As part of CPR, restoration of circulation starts with manual compression, but this produces only a fraction (5%) of the normal cerebral blood flow. Angiographic

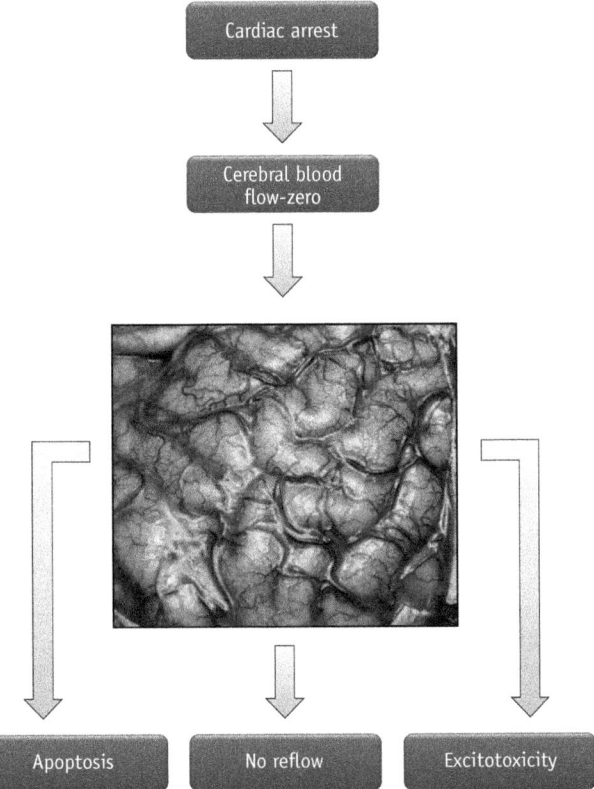

Figure 6.1 Mechanism of anoxic-ischemic injury to the brain.

and echocardiographic studies have shown that chest compression sets in motion an increase in intrathoracic pressure that causes blood to flow from the lung passively through the left side of the heart. The question of whether mechanical devices produce a better result was studied in the LUCAS in Cardiac Arrest randomized trial.[52] Mechanical chest compressions using a chest compression system (Physio-Control Inc., Lund, Sweden), in combination with defibrillation during ongoing compressions, did not improve survival or neurologic outcome when compared with manual CPR, although cerebral blood flow does seem significantly better with automated devices than with manual compression. Again, despite demonstrably better cortical cerebral blood flow in animal experiments, (Figure 6.2) the sad reality is that this does not translate to improvement in outcome. This device (and others) provides a positive intrathoracic pressure with chest compression, which causes a recoil—an important step that secures cardiac preload (this recoil is less common during manual compression). Defibrillation can occur with an operating device, freeing up one care provider. These devices can cause pancreatic injury, rib fracture, cardiac rupture, and esophageal rupture, but not as much as with manual resuscitation.[59]

The second core principle is that hypothermia may be the only effective therapy in patients who remain unresponsive after CPR. Targeted hypothermia does protect the brain but there is no evidence that hypothermia after percutaneous coronary intervention reduces myocardial infarct size.[23] Therapeutic hypothermia protocols have been developed and differ little from institution to institution. Generally speaking, there is an induction phase that provides temperature control

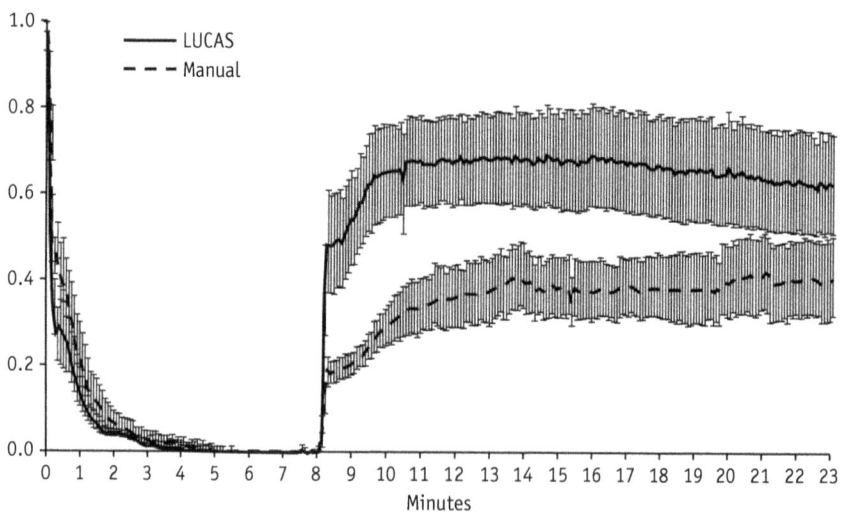

Figure 6.2 Cortical cerebral blood flow during manual cardiopulmonary resuscitation and resuscitation with the LUCAS system. Blood flow is represented as a fraction of the baseline flow value. (From Rubertsson and Karlsten[51] with permission.)

at target (34°C or 36°C) within 30–60 minutes.[44,61] Core cooling is best achieved with closed-loop devices rather than cooling blankets or ice packs. However, prehospital management may already have involved cooling with ice packs placed over the body. An infusion of cold (refrigerated) saline requires a central access line and is useful only as adjunct rather than initiation therapy. Shivering is anticipated with cooling and is treated with sedatives, opioids, or neuromuscular blocking agents. Vasopressors may be needed, but this may be primarily to treat cardiogenic shock resulting from myocardial pump failure. Hypotension and hyperglycemia can be injurious if not corrected promptly. The maintenance phase of therapeutic hypothermia is 24 hours, but rebound fever is currently treated with longer periods of hypothermia or normothermia.[33]

A third important core principle is that cardiac arrest and successful resuscitation may be followed by *postresuscitation disease*.[40,55] This rapidly progressing syndrome may determine outcome even more than brain injury does. These already comatose patients may need an aortic balloon pump next to multiple vasopressors and inotropes.Moreover there may be substantial liver and kidney injury and they may have become anuric requiring immediate dialysis. Very few family members would want to continue under these circumstances, and most physicians comply. This manifestation with different degrees of severity occurs in up to two thirds of patients who are resuscitated—in essence, it is "whole body ischemia" followed by reperfusion.[6] Timelines of different phases have been arbitrarily defined and some have suggested that interventions are most likely to work during the period from 20 minutes to 12 hours after cardiac arrest. The organs involved, beside the brain, are myocardium, kidney, liver, and adrenals. The systemic ischemia-reperfusion response results in impaired vasoregulation, increased coagulation, adrenal suppression, and abnormal oxygen delivery. Patients are hemodynamically labile, but even those with normal blood pressures have a poor cardiac index. Hypotension despite multiple vasopressors and inotropes could exacerbate brain ischemia because there is a severely impaired cerebral autoregulation. How much relative hypotension can be tolerated is not known. Therapeutic hypothermia (32°C–34°C) does decrease cardiac output by 24%–40%, but outcome does not seem to be compromised by the use of therapeutic hypothermia in patients with post–cardiac resuscitation syndrome.[43]

Renal replacement therapy and continuous dialysis for days to weeks may be needed. Most patients have impaired liver function tests, and repeated studies will show a rise of liver function tests in the thousands. There may be also thoracic injuries.[38] Oxygenation may be impaired because of pulmonary edema, which may be related to rib fractures or to management after a pneumothorax. Hyperoxemia (prolonged oxygenation with 100% inspired oxygen) may increase hospital mortality after cardiac arrest.[30]

Few consulting neurologists are fully aware that there is such a postresuscitation disease that involves cardiac stunning with hemodynamic instability and need for either artificial support through a balloon pump or ECMO. This intervention is needed because the stunning leads to marked reduction in myocardial function and exacerbates the problem.[49]

There has been an increased use of extracorporeal membrane oxygenation (ECMO), and it is useful to briefly review its principles. Basically, ECMO is a gas exchange pump (Figure 6.3). Deoxygenated blood passes through an oxygenator and is reinfused.[9] Blood drained from a vein and returned to a vein is called venovenous ECMO, but this does not require a pump. The rate of gas flow through the oxygenator and the blood flow rate essentially determine carbon dioxide removal.[10] In patients with poor cardiac function, a venoarterial circuit is needed. Patients with hypercapnic respiratory failure may be helped with a venovenous ECMO. The indication for ECMO is often also acute respiratory distress syndrome (ARDS) or pulmonary emboli followed by cardiac arrest, and ECMO may reduce mortality when compared with mechanical ventilation only.

Early studies have suggested improved neurologic outcome in patients with ventricular fibrillation or ventricular tachycardia who are treated with ECMO after CPR.[1,2,5,11,57,58] Hemorrhagic complications are common because of the need for anticoagulation to prevent thrombosis within the circuit and also because of thrombocytopenia. Limb ischemia and compartment syndrome are possible with venovenous ECMO. Guidelines for its use are available online.[13] The survival rate after CPR and ECMO is surprisingly good; a favorable outcome has been reported in approximately 80% of adults with in-hospital cardiac arrest. However, these

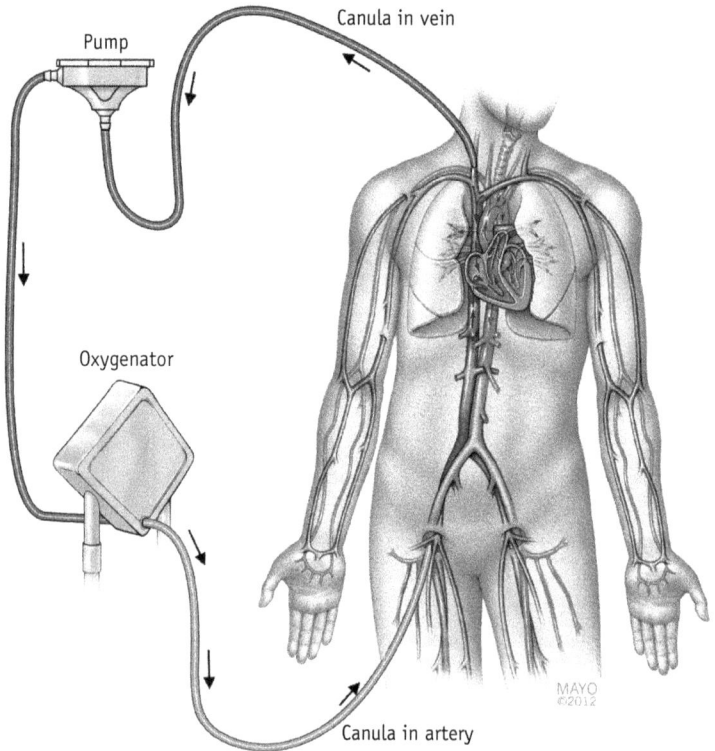

Figure 6.3 The extracorporeal membrane oxygenation device.

Table 6.1 **Clinical Syndromes After Anoxic-Ischemic Encephalopathy**

Clinical Syndrome	Mechanism	Outcome
"Man-in-the-barrel" syndrome	Bilateral watershed infarcts	Uncertain, may improve substantially
Parkinsonism	Infarcts in the striatum	Improvement possible
Action myoclonus	Cerebellar infarcts	Awake patients could improve with medication

studies were small, usually including not more than 20 patients. Poor predictors for poor outcome and mortality have included high increased lactate concentration and CPR duration longer than 30 minutes.

In careful assessment of the damage done, the most important core principle is to know why certain elements of the neurologic examination are important. A few simple facts are key here. Bilateral cortical injury may affect the motor response, changing it to no response to pain and flexor or extensor responses. Bilateral cortical injury and additional anoxic brainstem injury result in persistent extensor responses. When examined, it is likely that some brainstem reflexes are similarly involved, such as pupil responses to light and cornea reflexes to touch. Oculocephalic responses emerge in coma but may disappear with severe brainstem involvement. Inward and downward eye deviation does localize to the thalamus or mesencephalon. The gist of it all is that neurologic examination can establish the depth of coma and determine brainstem involvement as an indicator of far more severe anoxic-ischemic injury.[8,22,63]

Although a battery of tests—neuroimaging, electrophysiology, and laboratory studies—are available, none of them in themselves are sufficient to help in adequate prognostication. The principles of involvement of brainstem injury thus remains important.[16–18] Any patient who has a combination of two absent brainstem reflexes (e.g., pupil and cornea, pupil and oculocephalic responses) has a much lower probability of recovery. Motor responses—whether absent motor response or extensor posturing—by itself are not reliable early prognosticators. Occasionally, a clinical syndrome is noted, but most of the brain injury is diffusely spread out over the parieto-occipital cortex and knocks out multiple layers of cortex and thus not localized in certain parts of the brain (Table 6.1).

In Practice

In the United States, a patient who is comatose after cardiac arrest will likely be seen by a neurologist (hospitalist or neurointensivist). In Europe, a recent survey showed a neurologist appeared to be involved in about 25% and this observation is possibly responsible for a substantial uncertainty regarding neurological prognostication and decisions on level of care.[15]

The neurologist is asked to prognosticate and, increasingly, to comment on patients in more dire situations with complex support systems. Neurologists can participate in the discussion only if there is sufficient knowledge of the patient's medical and cardiac state. Foremost, if poor outcome is anticipated, any ICU or coronary care unit practice (as well as study groups reporting outcomes) will have to somehow define neurologic criteria for withdrawal of support. The most recent (and reasonable) proposal has come from the Targeted Temperature Management After Cardiac Arrest trial (Table 6.2) but it remains a difficult judgment call which cannot be simplified as a few rules.[42] Concerns remain about the accuracy of neurologic examination by non-neurologists, withdrawal of support without neurology consultation, withdrawal of support even during therapeutic hypothermia, and also physicians who cannot resist strong family preferences for premature withdrawal of care. All of these variables factor in—the proverbial elephant in the room—and determine outcome.

In 2006, the American Academy of Neurology formulated guidelines[63] for prognosis based on a critical selection of a small number of reliable studies. The conclusion was that after arrest, and without the use of active cooling, the presence of myoclonus status epilepticus and absence of pupil or corneal reflexes (or additional brainstem reflexes) clinically predict a poor outcome (nursing home care or worse) with sufficient certainty. If the patient has no N20 responses on SSEP, there is a fairly high likelihood that severe anoxic-ischemic injury has occurred. Serum neuron-specific enolase (NSE) may be increased (a baseline value or after repeated measurements), typically in patients who are more severely affected and

Table 6.2 **Criteria Allowing Withdrawal of Active Care in Patients with Persisting Coma After Cardiac Arrest, proposed by the Targeted Temperature Management After Cardiac Arrest Trial**

1. Advance directives.
2. The patient fullfills the clinical criteria of brain dead.
3. The patient develops severe myoclonus status in the first 24 hours after admission* and has a bilateral absence of N20 peaks on median nerve SSEP after rewarming.
4. At 72 hours after normothermia, the patient is persistingly comatose with no motor response or extensor responses and has bilateral absence of N20 peaks on median nerve SSEP.
5. At 72 hours after normothermia, the patient is in persisting coma with no motor responses or extensor responses and has a treatment-refractory status epilepticus.**
6. At 72 hours after normothermia, the patient is persistingly comatose with no motor responses or extensor responses and with no improvements 1 or 2 days later.

* Generalized myoclonic convulsions in face and extremities for 30 minutes or longer.

** Unresponsive to active treatment with sedatives and antiepileptics for at least 24 hours.

SSEP, somatosensory evoked potentials.

Adapted from Nielsen et al.[42]

are receiving multiple pressors or ECMO, but the prognostic value of this finding is far from accurate and marginal at best. NSE is a gamma isomer of enolase which is located in neurons. The usefulness of these biomarkers in prognostication may be more limited than electrophysiologic testing because none of these studies are automated, long laboratory turnaround times are impractical, and standardization of these immunometric assays is far from optimal. Therapeutic hypothermia has an effect on the metabolism and clearance of these biomarkers. Results of studies on the predictive value of NSE during or after hypothermia are conflicting, with some finding that NSE levels maintain prognostic accuracy and others finding the prognostic value to be reduced.[16] With a cutoff value of 33 µg/L for poor prognosis, false positive rates have been reported as high as 22%–29% after therapeutic hypothermia protocols. One study found that an NSE level as high as 79 µg/L is needed to achieve false positive rate of 0% for predicting unfavorable outcomes. Consistently high NSE values may have more predictive value[60] Differences in laboratory assays have made comparisons difficult, and there is no strict threshold level of NSE that can be recommended for use in prognostication after cardiac arrest and hypothermia until there is further research and standardization of these assays.

With the worldwide institution of therapeutic hypothermia, the absence of corneal reflexes is less reliable, as is motor response. Both responses are confounded by the use of sedatives or muscle relaxants during therapeutic hypothermia.[29] The practice has been to evaluate patients 72 hours after the ictus but with liberal use of sedation during hypothermia this time interval is not very useful. One study found that one third of patients treated with hypothermia awoke and had good neurologic outcome when assessed at 72 hours.[39] Recent advice to begin the 72-hour count at attainment of normothermia rather than at CPR also may not be sufficient particularly at institutions in which the sedoanalgesia practice is more aggressive.

Often, there are other findings that support the devastating nature of these manifestations, such as absence of N20 responses on SSEP recordings.[4,33] Burst-suppression EEG patterns are often misinterpreted as status epilepticus and are unnecessarily actively treated, only to find that seizures return after treatment is weaned. Most studies in survivors of CPR have found that patients who had "clinical seizures" were comatose and died from withdrawal of support. Moreover, myoclonus status epilepticus in combination with a markedly suppressed EEG remains one of the most important features that can help in determining poor prognosis. But, electrographic seizures on EEG again do not uniformly determine a poor outcome, and some patients benefit from brief treatment with a high dose of benzodiazepines or propofol. However, if seizures are seen while the patient is on a therapeutic hypothermia protocol, the chance of good outcome should be considered poor. It is well known that hypothermia reduces seizures, and breakthrough seizures would indicate a severely injured brain rather than seizures that require immediate control.

The ugly fact remains that some patients have had a long period of unwitnessed arrest and are admitted comatose with no motor response, with myoclonus status epilepticus, with tonic vertical gaze, and with test results that show abnormal

SSEPs, burst-suppression on EEG, and early brain edema on CT. This is usually associated with multiorgan failure, metabolic acidosis, anuria, tachypnea, and tachycardia, all pointing to a devastating injury. A poor outcome should come as no surprise to anyone.

ECMO can salvage patients, but in our experience, the likelihood of neurologic injury remains high, typically as a result of prolonged resuscitation.[37] Any patient who is evaluated on ECMO may have major confounders, such as marked hypoxemia, hyperglycemia, severe metabolic acidosis, and sodium abnormalities in both directions. Many patients have developed severe ARDS and their oxygenation is tenuous. When CT scans are done, cerebral infarcts or intracranial hemorrhage, or hemorrhage into the sulci, is often noted. In some patients, all brainstem reflexes disappear. They may need a formal brain death examination, which can be performed with some difficulty. A reliable apnea test is more complex and should require gradual increase of CO_2 rather than disconnection from the ventilator. Alternatively, a blood flow study may be

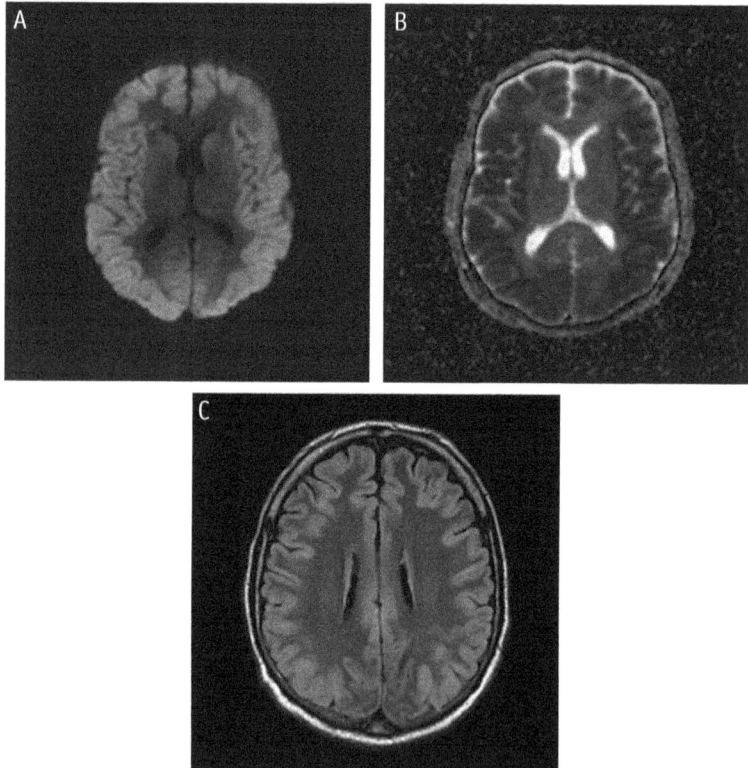

Figure 6.4 MRI images show injury indicating severe diffuse cortical necrosis: A, diffusion-weighted imaging (DWI); B, DWI with apparent diffusion coefficient mapping; and C, fluid-attenuated inversion recovery.

considered, but except for transcranial Doppler ultrasound, this is difficult because the patient is typically too unstable to be moved out of the cardiac ICU.

Magnetic resonance imaging (MRI) holds promise as an adjunct for determination of prognosis in comatose patients after cardiopulmonary arrest, but there are currently insufficient data to systematically guide prognostication with MRI. Diffusion-weighted imaging (DWI) is particularly sensitive to ischemia, and apparent diffusion coefficient values can provide a quantitative measure of injury (Figure 6.4). The current literature is limited by heterogeneity of MRI timing and patient selection bias. MRI parameters associated with poor outcome include widespread and persistent cortical DWI abnormalities. Moreover, although MRI results may be normal or indicate cortical injury on repeat studies, MRI cannot reliably and absolutely determine final outcome (persistent vegetative state, minimal conscious state, or fully aware severe disability). A normal MRI—like a normal SSEP—should not necessarily encourage prolonged aggressive support, and we have repeatedly seen patients with prolonged unconsciousness and normal MRIs (follow-up MRIs, months later, did eventually show diffuse atrophy).

A recent meta-analysis of 20 studies of outcome after therapeutic hypothermia concluded that many prognosticators from the pre-hypothermia era remained useful (Table 6.3)[21]. Therapeutic hypothermia may not be so "therapeutic," as we tend to believe and there are conflicting opinions, inviting skepticism.[19,20,25,35,49,50] In addition, "brain resuscitation" after cardiac arrest is an ambiguous term with little hard data to go by.[56] The question is, if targets of 33°C or 36°C did not make a difference, why would 37°C be harmful? Others feel 33°C should remain standard, arguing that one randomized study should not negate the results of 40 nonrandomized studies.[48] Major criticisms have included possible patient selection bias and rapid rewarming.

Table 6.3 **Precision of Diagnostic Tests for Predicting Poor Neurologic Outcome**

Diagnostic test	No. of patients tested	Sensitivity	Specificity	False positive rate
Corneal reflex	367	0.28	0.96	0.04
Pupillary reflex	438	0.24	0.98	0.02
Motor score (absent or posturing)	791	0.62	0.91	0.09
Myoclonic status	513	0.29	0.95	0.05
Unfavorable electroencephalogram	552	0.67	0.93	0.07
Somatosensory-evoked potentials (absent N20 responses)	620	0.43	0.90	0.03
Neuron-specific enolase (>33 µg/L)	507	0.05	0.88	0.12

Adapted from Golan et al.[21]

Another issue is whether hypothermia also protects other organs and whether organ dysfunction as a result of the ischemia-reperfusion response is reduced. This seems unlikely, and no apparent reduction has been shown in recent large trials. More recently, no benefit was found in an ambulance study with rapid cooling after successful resuscitation.[31]

To epitomize, we can expect that only a small fraction of comatose patients (<20%) will have reliable outcome predictors as evidenced by absence of some or all brainstem reflexes, persistent myoclonus, absence of cortical potentials on SSEP, and MRI proof of extensive cortical injury and that ICU care for these patients will likely be stopped or de-escalated. We can expect that patients who remain comatose with no motor responses or extensor responses and are critically ill from cardiac, liver, and renal failure will not be treated for very long. But how should families of patients who remain comatose for 2–3 weeks after resuscitation and therapeutic hypothermia but do not have these abnormal poor prognostic signs be approached? Specific time cutoffs are not useful because reliable data is not available. Some patients remain in a persistent vegetative state and then may or may not improve after 6 months. Failure to demonstrate blinking in response to threat, persistence of roving eye movements (or, worse, rapid ballistic movements), failure to fixate on approaching objects, and a nonlocalizing motor response should be considered sufficient information to predict long-term severe disability and need for 24-hour skilled nursing care.

Putting It All Together

- Therapeutic hypothermia works best in comatose patients after ventricular fibrillation or ventricular tachycardia and CPR.
- Prognostication may have changed in the current era of aggressive care.
- Brainstem injury after anoxia and myoclonus status epilepticus remain important prognosticators of poor outcome.
- Status epilepticus after anoxic-ischemic coma is difficult to treat effectively and thus often an indicator of severe cortical injury.
- Postresuscitation disease may already indicate poor outcome.

By the Way

- MRI in comatose patients after CPR is underutilized.
- CT scanning in comatose patients after CPR is usually normal and stays normal.
- Malignant EEG patterns are unusual and EEG mostly shows diffuse slowing and some reactivity.
- Most serum biomarkers are not clinically useful indicators of prognosis.

Comatose After CPR by the Numbers

- ~99% have a poor outcome if there is persistent myoclonus status
- ~99% have a poor outcome if there are absent pupil and corneal reflexes.
- ~95% have a poor outcome if there are absent cortical potentials on SSEP.
- ~80% have a poor outcome with burst-suppression or flat EEG.
- ~60% have a poor outcome with increased serum NSE level.

References

1. Abrams D, Combes A, Brodie D. Extracorporeal membrane oxygenation in cardiopulmonary disease in adults. *J Am Coll Cardiol* 2014;63:2769–2778.
2. Alsoufi B, Al-Radi OO, Nazer RI, et al. Survival outcomes after rescue extracorporeal cardiopulmonary resuscitation in pediatric patients with refractory cardiac arrest. *J Thorac Cardiovasc Surg* 2007;134:952–959, e952.
3. Ames A 3rd, Wright RL, Kowada M, Thurston JM, Majno G. Cerebral ischemia: II. The no-reflow phenomenon. *Am J Pathol* 1968;52:437–453.
4. Arch AE, Chiappa K, Greer DM. False positive absent somatosensory evoked potentials in cardiac arrest with therapeutic hypothermia. *Resuscitation* 2014;85:e97–e98.
5. Avalli L, Maggioni E, Formica F, et al. Favourable survival of in-hospital compared to out-of-hospital refractory cardiac arrest patients treated with extracorporeal membrane oxygenation: an Italian tertiary care centre experience. *Resuscitation* 2012;83:579–583.
6. Binks A, Nolan JP. Post-cardiac arrest syndrome. *Minerva Anestesiol* 2010;76:362–368.
7. Bottiger BW, Krumnikl JJ, Gass P, et al. The cerebral "no-reflow" phenomenon after cardiac arrest in rats: influence of low-flow reperfusion. *Resuscitation* 1997;34:79–87.
8. Bouwes A, Binnekade JM, Kuiper MA, et al. Prognosis of coma after therapeutic hypothermia: a prospective cohort study. *Ann Neurol* 2012;71:206–212.
9. Butt W, Maclaren G. Extracorporeal membrane oxygenation. *F1000Prime Rep* 2013;5:55.
10. Chauhan S, Subin S. Extracorporeal membrane oxygenation, an anesthesiologist's perspective: physiology and principles: Part 1. *Ann Card Anaesth* 2011;14:218–229.
11. Chen YS, Lin JW, Yu HY, et al. Cardiopulmonary resuscitation with assisted extracorporeal life-support versus conventional cardiopulmonary resuscitation in adults with in-hospital cardiac arrest: an observational study and propensity analysis. *Lancet* 2008;372:554–561.
12. Cronberg T, Brizzi M, Liedholm LJ, et al. Neurological prognostication after cardiac arrest: recommendations from the Swedish Resuscitation Council. *Resuscitation* 2013;84:867–872.
13. ELSO Guidelines for ECPR Cases v1.3, 2013. Extracorporeal Life Support Organization. https://www.elso.org/Resources/Guidelines.aspx. Accessed March 2015.
14. Fischer M, Hossmann KA. No-reflow after cardiac arrest. *Intensive Care Med* 1995;21:132–141.
15. Friberg H, Cronberg T, Dünser et al. Survey on current practices for neurological prognostication after cardiac arrest. *Resuscitation* 2015; in press.
16. Friberg H, Rundgren M, Westhall E, Nielsen N, Cronberg T. Continuous evaluation of neurological prognosis after cardiac arrest. *Acta Anaesthesiol Scand* 2013;57:6–15.
17. Fugate JE, Wijdicks EF, Mandrekar J, et al. Predictors of neurologic outcome in hypothermia after cardiac arrest. *Ann Neurol* 2010;68:907–914.
18. Fugate JE, Wijdicks EF, White RD, Rabinstein AA. Does therapeutic hypothermia affect time to awakening in cardiac arrest survivors? *Neurology* 2011;77:1346–1350.

19. Geocadin RG, Murthy SB. Prognostication following cardiac arrest: do we have our patients' safety in mind?. *Crit Care Med* 2014;42:1959–1961.
20. Geocadin RG Wijdicks EFM, Damian M, Mayer SA Dubinsky RM. Reducing brain injury following cardiopulmonary resuscitation. AAN guidelines to be published 2016.
21. Golan E, Barrett K, Alali AS, et al. Predicting neurologic outcome after targeted temperature management for cardiac arrest: systematic review and meta-analysis. *Crit Care Med* 2014;42:1919–1930.
22. Greer DM, Rosenthal ES, Wu O. Neuroprognostication of hypoxic-ischaemic coma in the therapeutic hypothermia era. *Nat Rev Neurol* 2014;10:190–203.
23. Grines CL. ICE-IT-1: intravascular cooling adjunctive to percutaneous coronary intervention for acute myocardial infarction (part 1): a preliminary review of results TCT 2004. Presented at the Transcatheter Therapeutics annual scientific session, Washington, DC, September 2004.
24. Hekmatpanah J. Cerebral blood flow dynamics in hypotension and cardiac arrest. *Neurology* 1973;23:174–180.
25. Hessel EA 2nd. Therapeutic hypothermia after in-hospital cardiac arrest: a critique. *J Cardiothorac Vasc Anesth* 2014;28:789–799.
26. Hogue N, Sabir H, Maes E et al. Validation of a neuropathology score using quantitative methods to evaluate brain injury in a pig model of hypoxia ischemia. *J Neurosci Meth* 2014;230:30–36.
27. Jo IJ, Shin TG, Sim MS, et al. Outcome of in-hospital adult cardiopulmonary resuscitation assisted with portable auto-priming percutaneous cardiopulmonary support. *Int J Cardiol* 2011;151:12–17.
28. Kagawa E, Dote K, Kato M, et al. Should we emergently revascularize occluded coronaries for cardiac arrest? Rapid-response extracorporeal membrane oxygenation and intra-arrest percutaneous coronary intervention. *Circulation* 2012;126:1605–1613.
29. Kamps MJ, Horn J, Oddo M, et al. Prognostication of neurologic outcome in cardiac arrest patients after mild therapeutic hypothermia: a meta-analysis of the current literature. *Intensive Care Med* 2013;39:1671–1682.
30. Kilgannon JH, Jones AE, Shapiro NI, et al. Association between arterial hyperoxia following resuscitation from cardiac arrest and in-hospital mortality. *JAMA* 2010;303:2165–2171.
31. Kim F, Nichol G, Maynard C, et al. Effect of prehospital induction of mild hypothermia on survival and neurological status among adults with cardiac arrest: a randomized clinical trial. *JAMA* 2014;311:45–52.
32. Le Guen M, Nicolas-Robin A, Carreira S, et al. Extracorporeal life support following out-of-hospital refractory cardiac arrest. *Crit Care* 2011;15:R29.
33. Leithner C, Ploner CJ, Hasper D, Storm C. Does hypothermia influence the predictive value of bilateral absent N2O after cardiac arrest? *Neurology* 2010;74:965–969.
34. Lemiale V, Huet O, Vigue B, et al. Changes in cerebral blood flow and oxygen extraction during post-resuscitation syndrome. *Resuscitation* 2008;76:17–24.
35. Little NE, Feldman EL. Therapeutic hypothermia after cardiac arrest without return of consciousness: skating on thin ice. *JAMA Neurol* 2014;71:823–824.
36. Liu S, Connor J, Peterson S, Shuttleworth CW, Liu KJ. Direct visualization of trapped erythrocytes in rat brain after focal ischemia and reperfusion. *J Cereb Blood Flow Metab* 2002; 22:1222–1230.
37. Mateen FJ, Muralidharan R, Shinohara RT, et al. Neurological injury in adults treated with extracorporeal membrane oxygenation. *Arch Neurol* 2011;68:1543–1549.
38. Miller AC, Rosati SF, Suffredini AF, Schrump DS. A systematic review and pooled analysis of CPR-associated cardiovascular and thoracic injuries. *Resuscitation* 2014;85:724–731.
39. Mulder M, Gibbs HG, Smith SW, et al. Awakening and withdrawal of life-sustaining treatment in cardiac arrest survivors treated with therapeutic hypothermia. *Crit Care Med* 2014;42:2493–2499.
40. Negovsky VA. Postresuscitation disease. *Crit Care Med* 1988;16:942–946.

41. Nielsen N, Wetterslev J, al-Subaie N, et al. Target Temperature Management after out-of-hospital cardiac arrest: a randomized, parallel-group, assessor-blinded clinical trial—rationale and design. *Am Heart J* 2012;163:541–548.
42. Nielsen N, Wetterslev J, Cronberg T, et al. Targeted temperature management at 33 degrees C versus 36 degrees C after cardiac arrest. *N Engl J Med* 2013;369:2197–2206.
43. Oksanen T, Skrifvars M, Wilkman E, et al. Postresuscitation hemodynamics during therapeutic hypothermia after out-of-hospital cardiac arrest with ventricular fibrillation: a retrospective study. *Resuscitation* 2014;85:1018–1024.
44. Perman SM, Goyal M, Neumar RW, Topjian AA, Gaieski DF. Clinical applications of targeted temperature management. *Chest* 2014;145:386–393.
45. Polderman KH. Application of therapeutic hypothermia in the ICU: opportunities and pitfalls of a promising treatment modality. Part 1: indications and evidence. *Intensive Care Med* 2004;30:556–575.
46. Polderman KH. Mechanisms of action, physiological effects, and complications of hypothermia. *Crit Care Med* 2009;37:S186–S202.
47. Polderman KH, Herold I. Therapeutic hypothermia and controlled normothermia in the intensive care unit: practical considerations, side effects, and cooling methods. *Crit Care Med* 2009;37:1101–1120.
48. Polderman KH, Varon J. We should not abandon therapeutic cooling after cardiac arrest. *Crit Care* 2014;18:130.
49. Rolston DM, Lee J. March 2014 Annals of Emergency Medicine Journal Club: is it still cool to cool? Interpreting the latest hypothermia for cardiac arrest trial. *Ann Emerg Med* 2014;63:368–369.
50. Rossetti AO, Oddo M, Logroscino G, Kaplan PW. Prognostication after cardiac arrest and hypothermia: a prospective study. *Ann Neurol* 2010;67:301–307.
51. Rubertsson S, Karlsten R. Increased cortical cerebral blood flow with LUCAS: a new device for mechanical chest compressions compared to standard external compressions during experimental cardiopulmonary resuscitation. *Resuscitation* 2005;65:357–363.
52. Rubertsson S, Lindgren E, Smekal D, et al. Mechanical chest compressions and simultaneous defibrillation vs conventional cardiopulmonary resuscitation in out-of-hospital cardiac arrest: the LINC randomized trial. *JAMA* 2014;311:53–61.
53. Sandroni C, Cavallaro F, Callaway CW, et al. Predictors of poor neurological outcome in adult comatose survivors of cardiac arrest: a systematic review and meta-analysis. Part 1: patients not treated with therapeutic hypothermia. *Resuscitation* 2013;84:1310–1323.
54. Sandroni C, Cavallaro F, Callaway CW, et al. Predictors of poor neurological outcome in adult comatose survivors of cardiac arrest: a systematic review and meta-analysis. Part 2: patients treated with therapeutic hypothermia. *Resuscitation* 2013;84:1324–1338.
55. Sasson C, Rogers MA, Dahl J, Kellermann AL. Predictors of survival from out-of-hospital cardiac arrest: a systematic review and meta-analysis. *Circ Cardiovasc Qual Outcomes* 2010;3:63–81.
56. Schneider A, Bottiger BW, Popp E. Cerebral resuscitation after cardiocirculatory arrest. *Anesth Analg* 2009;108:971–979.
57. Shin TG, Choi JH, Jo IJ, et al. Extracorporeal cardiopulmonary resuscitation in patients with inhospital cardiac arrest: a comparison with conventional cardiopulmonary resuscitation. *Crit Care Med* 2011;39:1–7.
58. Shin TG, Jo IJ, Sim MS, et al. Two-year survival and neurological outcome of in-hospital cardiac arrest patients rescued by extracorporeal cardiopulmonary resuscitation. *Int J Cardiol* 2013;168:3424–3430.
59. Smekal D, Johansson J, Huzevka T, Rubertsson S. No difference in autopsy detected injuries in cardiac arrest patients treated with manual chest compressions compared with mechanical compressions with the LUCAS device: a pilot study. *Resuscitation* 2009;80:1104–1107.

60. Stammet P, Collignon O, Hassager C et al. Neuron-Specific Enolase as a Predictor of Death or Poor Neurological Outcome After Out-of-Hospital Cardiac Arrest and Targeted Temperature Management at 33°C and 36°C. *J Am Coll Cardiol* 2015;65:2104–2114.
61. Sunde K, Pytte M, Jacobsen D, et al. Implementation of a standardised treatment protocol for post resuscitation care after out-of-hospital cardiac arrest. *Resuscitation* 2007; 73:29–39.
62. Warner DS, James ML, Laskowitz DT, Wijdicks EF. Translational research in acute central nervous system injury: lessons learned and the future. *JAMA Neurol* 2014;71:1311–1318.
63. Wijdicks EF, Hijdra A, Young GB, Bassetti CL, Wiebe S. Practice parameter: prediction of outcome in comatose survivors after cardiopulmonary resuscitation (an evidence-based review). Report of the Quality Standards Subcommittee of the American Academy of Neurology. *Neurology* 2006;67:203–210.

7

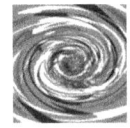

Acquired Weakness in the Intensive Care Unit

After a while, any critical illness leads to "weakness" and marked deconditioning.[41] Some patients—after weeks of treatment—can hardly stand and walk in the intensive care unit (ICU), mostly because of poor stamina along with poor lung and cardiac reserve. Muscle bulk shrinks rapidly during immobilization and even more rapidly in heavily sedated patients, and certainly in those who are pharmaceutically paralyzed. When muscles are fully inactive, they break down through a mechanism of proteolysis due to protease activation. This may be more noticeable in patients who are admitted with an already frail body habitus. The ultimate question here is to determine whether it represents profound muscle bulk loss after a life-threatening illness or a separate pathophysiologic process directed toward the nerves and muscles—and how much does it matter to know these precise details in a patient with flaccid limbs? To differentiate the two conditions, clinically and electrophysiologically, a neurologist is required.

The prevalence of *ICU-acquired weakness* (a new, broader term and less specific than critical illness polyneuromyopathy) is high among survivors of critical illness and increases as more patients survive multiorgan failure, sepsis, and other fulminant infections.[7,17,20,22,39] Working toward ICU discharge is often a long process, with gradual weaning of the ventilator and motor and gait rehabilitation. Many patients are permanently changed, and more than 50% of those in this state do not return to work.[19]

Serious damage to the nerves and muscles—and likely both—can occur in these very sick patients. The risk to be affected may approach 90% in patients with severe sepsis that has led to organ failure.[7,24,25,28] Very few patients develop profound weakness if there have not been clinical signs of sepsis. Again, the impact of this weakness on recovery is substantial, and among patients who survive septic shock—and there are not many—this handicap is a major part of their reduced quality of life.

Just as the definition of critical illness is arbitrary, so is the term ICU-acquired weakness. Moreover, management of critical illness polyneuropathy or critical illness polyneuromyopathy (both abbreviated in this chapter as CIP) starts with understanding the condition, and that is where the problem begins. Questions neurologists have to ask themselves in this situation are the following: Is this patient truly weak from a new neurologic disorder or more likely deconditioned? Is there a neurogenic component to failure to wean off the ventilator? Is the weakness of peripheral or central origin, and could spinal cord damage play a role? Is the weakness part of a more chronic systemic illness that might have predisposed the patient to sepsis? What brought the patient to the ICU in the first place, and might there be evidence of a prior unappreciated neuromuscular disorder? This chapter provides a full overview on how to approach a patient who is weak and wilted after a critical illness but may have a significant neurologic disorder.

Principles

Apart from understanding the underlying mechanism, the first core principle is to retrace the motor unit and determine systematically if the severe weakness is caused by a disorder of the spinal cord, motor neuron, plexus, peripheral nerve, neuromuscular junction (NMJ), or skeletal muscle. This can be determined by a comprehensive neurologic examination, which should include inspection for fasciculations or myokymias, assessment of the pattern of weakness (distal or proximal), tone (flaccid or spastic), and detection of other findings (face, eye, and tongue movements) suggesting an underlying neurologic disorder. If feasible sensory findings are important to consider. Still, most patients seen in the ICU have flaccid, immobile extremities with normal cranial nerve function.

Another core principle is to look for a specific neuromuscular disorder (Table 7.1). Although intensivists "hope" the neurologist will find one, this is highly unlikely, and findings on examination are typically much more unexciting and less urgent. The two most dramatic finds in my personal encounters are patients with acute respiratory failure and severe quadriparesis who have amyotrophic lateral sclerosis (ALS), but at that stage, tongue fasciculations are common and easily detected. Not infrequently, I have seen respiratory weakness in patients with myotonic dystrophy, in whom myotonia may easily be elicited by tapping on the thenar muscles.

Most neurologists will expect CIP or critical illness myopathy or both. One could argue that this is, in fact, the most common cause of weakness in the ICU. But there is no good understanding of what factor or factors are responsible for the emergence of CIP. Who are these patients in the greater scheme of things? Could it be that over the years we became complacent in attributing weakness to CIP in most cases? CIP is exclusively seen in patients who have been mechanically ventilated and immobilized for some time (Figure 7.1).

It is not clear whether CIP is a disorder in its own right. Initially, there was a major emphasis on malnutrition, use of antibiotics, neuromuscular blocking agents, and hyperglycemia, but these are derangements that are typically seen with any critical illness.[35,45,50] Other risk factors are dialysis during critical illness, use of pressors, duration of mechanical ventilation, and multiorgan failure and sepsis. The most important clinical circumstance is the link between CIP, sepsis, multiorgan failure, and prolonged stay in the ICU. One theory is that there is diffuse tissue hypoxemia in the setting of shock and acute respiratory distress syndrome that leads to axonal injury. Studies on hyperglycemia in a post hoc analysis found that maintenance of blood glucose levels between 80 and 110 mg/dL (strict control) reduced CIP by almost 50%; but, although

Table 7.1 **Neuromuscular Conditions Causing Generalized Weakness in the Intensive Care Unit**

Muscle diseases
- Critical illness myopathy
- Inflammatory myopathies (polymyositis, dermatomyositis)
- Hypokalemic myopathy
- Rhabdomyolysis
- Muscular dystrophies
- Myotonic dystrophy
- Mitochondrial myopathies
- Acid maltase deficiency

Neuromuscular Junction disorders
- Myasthenia gravis
- Neuromuscular blocking agent–induced weakness
- Antibiotic-induced myasthenia gravis
- Organophosphorus poisoning
- Snake bite
- Insect/marine toxins
- Lambert–Eaton myasthenic syndrome
- Congenital myasthenic syndromes
- Hypermagnesemia
- Botulism
- Tick paralysis

Peripheral neuropathies
- Guillain–Barré syndrome
- Chronic idiopathic demyelinating polyneuropathy
- Critical illness polyneuropathy
- Toxic neuropathy
- Vasculitic neuropathy
- Porphyric neuropathy
- Diphtheria
- Lymphoma
- Cytomegalovirus-related polyradiculoneuropathy

Anterior horn cell disorders
- Amyotrophic lateral sclerosis
- Paraneoplastic motor neuron disease
- West Nile virus infection
- Acute poliomyelitis
- Spinal muscular atrophy

Spinal cord disorders
- Trauma
- Hematoma
- Spinal cord infarction
- Epidural abscess
- Demyelination (multiple sclerosis, Devic's disease, acute disseminated encephalomyelitis, transverse myelitis)
- Infective myelitis (coxsackievirus A and B, cytomegalovirus, *Mycoplasma*, *Legionella*, herpes zoster)
- Paralytic rabies ("dumb rabies")

Adapted from Maramattom and Wijdicks.[35]

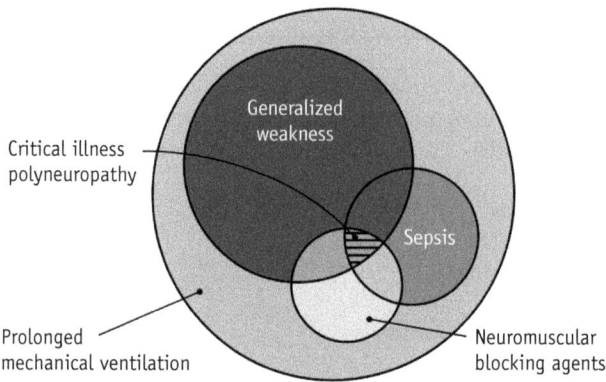

Figure 7.1 The scope of the problem and the population in whom critical illness polyneuropathy may be expected.

this is potentially of interest, strict control of glucose has increased mortality and thus the observation—even if correct—is irrelevant. Others have suggested a mitochondrial dysfunction in axons resulting from hypoxemia or from damage caused by inflammatory markers such as interleukins, tumor necrosis factor, platelet activating factor, leukotrienes, and thromboxane among many others. One group identified a toxin of low molecular weight that was not further characterized, and there has not been a confirmatory study.[8]

A basic question is whether the neurons are part of the inflammatory assault on organs or whether there is a more specific immunologic response toward the axons or myelin sheath. One hypothesis that may get traction is endothelial cell activation by inflammatory mediators (complement factors, adhesion molecules, antigen-presenting molecules). Increased vascular permeability may result in edema and ischemia. This microvascular ischemia of nerves, together with dysfunction of sodium channels and injury to mitochondria, has been proposed as a possible mechanism of nerve and muscle injury (Figure 7.2).[2,11,25,49]

Cachexia—now considered a metabolic syndrome associated with increased inflammatory markers (C-reactive protein and interleukin 6)—may at least partly explain critical illness myopathy. Muscle protein synthesis may be reduced by the presence of proinflammatory cytokines in sepsis and immobility may additionally contribute.[23,44] Most fascinating is the link between gut microorganisms and muscle, suggesting that amino acid availability can change muscle physiology.[3] This could link muscle wasting to sepsis. Similarly, atrophy and weakness in the diaphragm causing respiratory failure can be linked to cachexia of prolonged critical illness. Loss of both type I and type II muscle fibers has been found, but more likely there is structural disorganization causing loss in contractility.[43] Truth be told, reduced muscle activity and protein–calorie malnutrition causing very thin muscles should not necessarily reduce strength.

It has been known since the first description that use of neuromuscular blocking agents is correlated with acquired weakness, particularly if combined with high-dose intravenous corticosteroids. Muscle biopsies have found denervated muscle fibers,

Acquired Weakness in the Intensive Care Unit   97

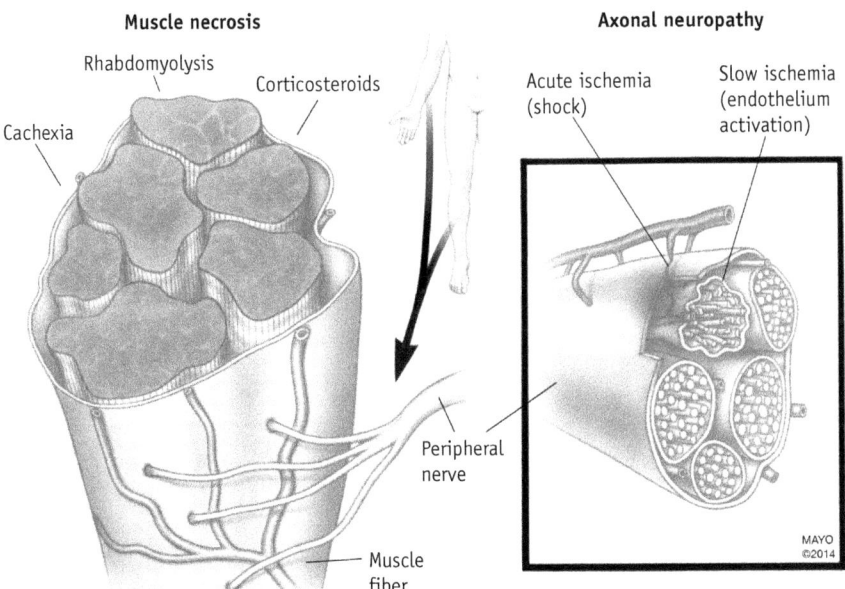

Figure 7.2 Proposed mechanisms of injury in polyneuropathy and myopathy of critical illness.

myosin filament destruction, and acute necrosis in patients receiving high-dose corticosteroids. Glucocorticoids do act on the NMJ and have been shown to decrease potentials at this junction; therefore, they also inactivate sodium channels and may induce loss of thick filaments. Furthermore, there is evidence that glucocorticoids inhibit protein synthesis, leading to muscle catabolism. Each of these explanations is insufficient to explain the pathophysiologic mechanism. Although myopathic changes may predominate on electrophysiologic testing, the nature of this myopathy is not completely clear. Biopsies have described several types of abnormalities in acquired weakness: predominant necrosis, muscle loss from likely rhabdomyolysis, and loss of thick filaments; however, this further characterization does nothing to explain its appearance. There is a known link of corticosteroids with acute myopathy in aggressive treatment of status asthmaticus, but often corticosteroids cannot be implicated in these patients.

Neuromuscular blocking agents play an important role in early and late manifestations of neuromuscular weakness in the ICU. As mentioned in Chapter 1, depolarizing NMJ blockers (i.e., succinyl choline) bind to receptors and depolarize the muscle membrane, opening the channel and stopping the activity. This drug cannot be reversed, and its slow breakdown leads to slow recovery of muscle strength. Non-depolarizing blockers bind to receptors but without channel opening, basically competing with acetylcholine. It can be easily understood why neostigmine works in this situation (it inhibits breakdown of acetylcholine by choline esterase) and thus its increased availability at the receptor (Figure 7.3). Prolonged weakness has been linked to these long-acting

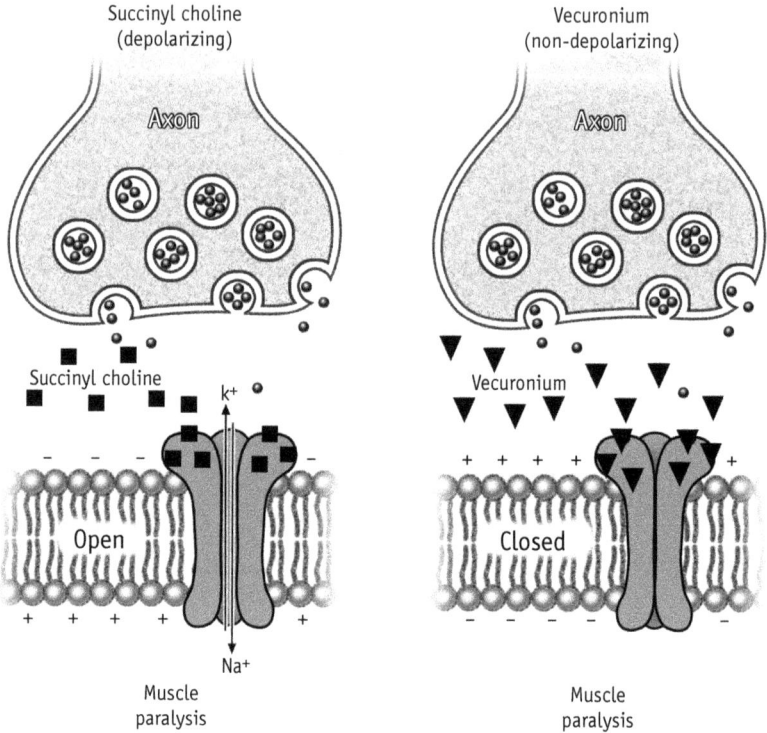

Figure 7.3 Effects of succinyl choline and vecuronium at the neuromuscular junction (see text for explanation).

drugs, but there is little information about shorter-acting agents such as atracurium and rocuronium. It can be said that 24–48 hours of administration of NMJ blockers will have an effect on muscle, but this is an unstudied topic with no explanatory pathologic substrate found on biopsies (e.g., inflammatory cell clusters, some muscle necrosis).

Loss of muscle mass is expected in immobilized critically ill patients because inactivity induces muscle unloading. Nutritional deficiency may also contribute to loss of muscle bulk when a catabolic state is not balanced by high caloric intake. This state can be expected in any patient with sepsis, trauma, burns, or previous malnourishment due to alcohol or drug abuse. Specific vitamin deficiencies have not consistently been shown to produce myopathic changes on biopsy examinations except for vitamin E in malabsorption syndromes. Parenteral nutrition in most patients is usually balanced with the use of well-tested formulas in the hospital, but when catabolism strikes, and is overwhelmingly severe, patients may still attain a negative nitrogen balance. Prolonged immobilization may lead to muscle wasting due to depressed insulin-induced glucose transport.

Disuse of skeletal muscle rapidly produces atrophy. Muscle biopsy shows intact architecture, little change in type I muscle fibers, and mostly degeneration of type II fibers. When muscle biopsies are performed in critically ill patients, muscle atrophy is noted within 10 days after ICU admission and in almost 70% of the patients in later biopsies. Some abnormalities may be seen in clusters, but type grouping, as in neurogenic disease, is not evident. Prolonged immobilization of limbs in patients with neuromuscular blockade may produce some pressure necrosis in some muscles, but not enough to explain the dramatic loss.

Rhabdomyolysis may be a cause of weakness in critically ill patients. The prevalence of rhabdomyolysis is not known, but it may be much higher than appreciated because its triggers are so common in critical illness. The most common causes are probably trauma and ischemia from arterial occlusion. Rhabdomyolysis may be severe with acute poisonings and illicit drug use when they contain sympathomimetic effects.

Most patients with extensive rhabdomyolysis have considerable muscle weakness and pain when tested. Biceps, quadriceps, and gastrocnemius muscles are tender on palpation and may appear swollen. Rapid resolution of weakness and decrease in the level of creatine kinase (CK), often from initial serum levels of about 10,000 IU, are expected within 2–3 days. The initial spike in CK may go unnoticed, and only muscle biopsy may be able to prove the diagnosis. Myoglobinuria can be seen, but this requires marked loss of muscle fibers.

In Practice

Acquired weakness in the ICU is best defined as weakness that develops during the onset of critical illness and involves both proximal and distal muscles—it is profound, symmetric, flaccid, and there is sparing of muscles innervated by the cranial nerves. Typically, the Medical Research Council (MRC) score is less than 2 for most muscle groups and the patient is fully dependent on mechanical ventilation and tracheostomized.

Studies reviewing the spectrum of neuromuscular weakness usually focus on patients who were referred for electrophysiologic studies, rather than on all patients in the ICU. It appears that myopathy is found in 46%, peripheral neuropathy in 28%, motor neuron disease in 7%, and myasthenic syndromes in 3% in such studies. However, these frequencies do not reflect our experiences at Mayo Clinic hospitals, where we almost always find a combination of axonal and muscle injury. Part of the problem is patients' comorbidities, including a very high prevalence of type II diabetes which may be associated with previously underlying polyneuropathy. Rarely, and not more than once or twice a year, a neurologic disorder is discovered.

The first approach to evaluating weakness in the ICU is to classify and categorize the findings on examination. One useful way to standardize evaluations is to use the mnemonic MUSCLES (Figure 7.4).[48]

Examination is best documented by the MRC score.[16] If the patient has flaccid quadriparesis, one often cannot tell whether the problem is in spinal cord, muscle, or nerve. Tendon reflexes may not be helpful either, if the injury is fairly recent. Often all that is found is weakness of limbs and not of facial, laryngeal, or neck muscles. Severe muscle wasting is seen, with prominence of bones and tendons that are normally surrounded by muscle bulk. In many patients, the tendon reflexes and sensation for touch, pinprick, and proprioception are preserved arguing, at least clinically, against nerve injury, but not when nerve conduction studies are done. Often, clues

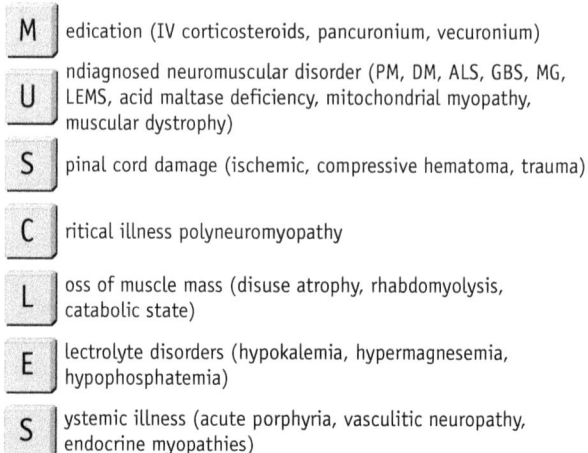

Figure 7.4 MUSCLES mnemonic. ALS, amyotrophic lateral sclerosis; DM, diabetes mellitus; GBS, Guillain–Barré syndrome; LEMS, Lambert–Eaton myasthenic syndrome; MG, myasthenia gravis; PM, polymyositis.

can be found that point toward no neurologic disease but purely toward debilitation from prolonged ICU stay.[14]

Myopathies typically produce more proximal muscle weakness (e.g., quadriceps), and neuropathies more distal muscle weakness. Neuromuscular weakness associated with NMJ abnormalities produce fatigable weakness (e.g., myasthenia gravis) or flaccid weakness (e.g., from organophosphates).

Vasculitic neuropathy causes a multifocal sensorimotor neuropathy, often footdrop. There is pain, and onset is abrupt. It should be considered with the more frequent systemic vasculitic syndromes (Wegener's granulomatosis, systemic lupus erythematous, and polyarteritis nodosa). These disorders may have been transferred to the ICU as a result of medical complications or as a result of a complication of immunosuppression.

Myopathies associated with multisystemic illness should be recognized and usually are seen with rare disorders such as systemic amyloidosis. Myopathic disorders may produce myotonia (delayed relaxation of muscle after percussion or voluntary contraction), muscle tenderness (rhabdomyolysis), and skin lesions. Severe necrotic myopathy may occur in patients with brittle diabetes. Dermatomyositis has been associated with a large number of cancers. The rash of dermatomyositis is periorbital and purple. Rashes over the knuckles (Gottron's sign) may be seen. Critical illness myopathy is thus a diagnosis of exclusion.[29]

Disorders of the NMJ are not commonly found in the ICU unless a myasthenia gravis is detected. Several cancers can cause paraneoplastic syndromes, but small cell lung cancer has an association with Lambert–Eaton myasthenic syndrome. There is marked weakness of proximal muscles, causing difficulty with rising from a sitting position; often, there is prominence of autonomic symptoms such as dry mouth, dry eyes, and postural hypotension.

Polyneuropathies may or may not have cranial nerve involvement. Cranial nerve involvement should point to Guillain–Barré syndrome (GBS), botulism, or West Nile virus infection, but these are highly uncommon explanations.

The electrophysiologic study should involve at least two motor and two sensory nerve studies and repetitive nerve stimulation at 2–3 Hz.[26,37] In most patients, there will be no NMJ transmission deficit (its presence with normal compound muscle action potentials [CMAPs] denotes myasthenia gravis; with low CMAPs, botulism or Lambert–Eaton syndrome). NMJ transmission disorder can be caused iatrogenically by the use of NMJ blockers, but electromyography (EMG) or nerve conduction studies should not be performed if these drugs have been recently stopped. The next step is to look at the duration of motor unit potentials: short (indicating severe myopathy, either inflammatory, necrotizing, or toxic) or long (motor neuron disease or long-standing polyneuropathy such as in diabetes). Motor unit potentials of normal duration may still point to a myopathy if direct stimulation of the muscle is absent.[42]

The presence of abnormal sensory nerve action potentials (SNAP) and compound muscle action potentials (CMAP) and fibrillation potentials points to an axonal polyneuropathy (CIP or severe axonal GBS). In CIP, the finding of low CMAPs has been described as early as 3 days after onset of sepsis.[21,27-30] The abnormalities of nerve function correlate strongly with severity of critical illness and time spent in the ICU. Similar findings of fibrillation potentials and reduced motor unit recruitment can be found in the diaphragm, but many patients on mechanical ventilators already have diaphragmatic atrophy (within days on assist-control modes).[31,32] Others have suggested the use of pulmonary function tests or ultrasound of the diaphragm to monitor for ICU-acquired weakness, but there is little useful data published.[46]

There are several concerns when interpreting nerve conduction velocity and EMG results. First, the CMAP amplitude may be reduced because of tissue edema. Abnormal coagulation in a critically ill patient may make EMG problematic, although it is not expected that a single needle will cause a significant hematoma. (There is no reason to hold anticoagulation, but an international normalized ratio less than 3 is preferred.[12])

One recent study used a cutoff value for the extensor digitorum brevis peroneal CMAP amplitude of less than 0.65 mV for diagnosis of ICU-acquired weakness; this resulted in a sensitivity of 94% and a specificity of 74%.[37] High diagnostic accuracy of the sural SNAP amplitude was also found, but the study identified a lower cutoff value for ICU patients than for healthy controls.

In summary, electrophysiologic features of critical illness myopathy seems apparent with reduced CMAP amplitude, short-duration units, and early recruitment; whereas in CIP, one may be able to find reduced CMAP and SNAP amplitudes with decreased recruitment, fibrillation potentials, and positive sharp waves. Lack of direct stimulation of the muscle is diagnostic for critical illness myopathy. Sensory potentials can be reduced in CIP, but this occurs more often in patients who have an underlying systemic illness such as diabetes mellitus. The SNAPs in ALS are normal. Patients with motor neuron disease have polyphasic waveforms with late components, poor recruitment, and widespread fibrillation and fasciculations. In all patients, it is best to specifically look for a possible decremental response which may indicate myasthenia gravis or a myasthenic syndrome (a progressive decrement pattern at low rates of repetitive nerve stimulation argues more for a myasthenic syndrome).

Clinical evaluation should probably include measurement of serum CK concentrations, but the initial spike—if any—may have passed and the values may now be normal. Biopsy of muscle may be considered, as well as nerve biopsy, but many of these biopsies are nonspecific and they often show type 2 denervation. In early development, muscle ultrasound has been used to detect critical illness neuromyopathy fairly easy in a large proportion of patients.[13] Muscle echogenicity in the early course of sepsis may be detected, but the correlation with EMG and nerve conduction studies is not known.

A commonly asked question is whether a chronically ventilated patient who cannot be weaned off the ventilator has a phrenic nerve injury. Off the ventilator, breathing is markedly asynchronous and paradoxical due to marked diaphragmatic atrophy and dysfunction. Phrenic nerve studies may be difficult to reliably interpret, and needle examination of the diaphragm is often abnormal with fibrillations and reduced recruitment in any patient with prolonged mechanical ventilation. Ultrasound of the chest may be helpful in demonstrating the degree of dysfunction.[5] Practically speaking, it may be difficult to attribute failure of weaning with certainty to phrenic nerve involvements and it is far most likely that dyssynchronous breathing is a result of marked diaphragmatic atrophy.

The best management of CIP and flaccid quadriparesis is aggressive, early physical therapy, but there are no established rehabilitation programs.[36] Early mobilization and physical therapy using passive range of motion are likely important.[1,6,10,15,33,38,40] Mobilization in the ICU is now commonplace for patients who are able to ambulate for at least 100 feet.[1] Adequate nutrition is important, and reassessment and supplementation of caloric intake and other elements may be needed.[9] There is insufficient evidence to show that intravenous immunoglobulin (IVIG) or plasma exchange improves outcome, and initial attempts have been unsuccessful.

Results of long-term outcome studies have been quite disturbing, with a large proportion of patients who survive being disabled by CIP. In general, patients with an isolated critical illness myopathy have a better prognosis than those who develop CIP alone or in combination with critical illness myopathy. Most recoveries occur early in patients with critical illness myopathy, usually within the first 3-6 months; whereas patients with a combination of myopathy and neuropathy may require at least 12 months for further recovery. A recently completed study of detailed muscle testing in 415 patients with prolonged ICU stay found weakness in half of the patients. There was a trend in these patients toward common poor nutritional scores, more sepsis, and longer corticosteroid treatment.[17] Mortality was higher in patients with persistent weakness. IVIG did not improve outcome in several studies.[4,47]

So where does this information leave us? Unfortunately, the patient with ICU-acquired weakness can be described as frail, barely survived, barely ready to leave the ICU, unable to ambulate due to poor strength, and unable to safely swallow due to dyssynchronous breathing or other factors.[19,34] It would be overly simplistic to attribute poor outcome (or mortality) to ICU-acquired weakness; most likely, it is just another manifestation of a major illness in a patient with severe preexisting comorbidity. Many patients have cardiac failure, pulmonary failure, and renal failure, making every step during mobilization a major exercise. Moreover, balance difficulties from poor preexisting or acquired proprioception increase the risk of fall and injury.[18] Once a major neurologic disorder has been excluded (the majority of cases), rehabilitation to improve a severely deconditioned state may not be possible, and nursing home placement may be more realistic—at least for some time. Now that patients more frequently survive critical illness, we may have to face the consequences of our aggressive management or try in some way to improve their quality of life with small interventions.

Putting It All Together

- Not all weakness in the ICU is a result of polyneuropathy or myopathy.
- EMG overestimates nerve and muscle injuries.
- Many patients on mechanical ventilators develop atrophy and major dysfunction of the diaphragm, resulting in paradoxical breathing.
- Weakness in the ICU may be caused by an unrecognized neurologic disorder or syndrome.

By the Way

- Early mobility and avoiding heavy sedation is the best preventive measure.
- Aggressive control of hyperglycemia could reduce the frequency of CIP.
- The effect of adequate nutrition on CIP is unknown.
- Phrenic nerve involvement in CIP is uncommon.

Critical Illness polyneuropathy and myopathy by the Numbers

- ~70% of patients with multiorgan failure and sepsis develop CIP.
- ~50% of patients with quadriparesis have EMG evidence of myopathy.
- ~50% of patients with CIP are quadriparetic for 1–5 years.
- ~30% of patients with CIP are quadriplegic for 1 year.
- ~10% of patients with critical illness myopathy are still weak after 1 year.

References

1. Bailey P, Thomsen GE, Spuhler VJ, et al. Early activity is feasible and safe in respiratory failure patients. *Crit Care Med* 2007;35:139–145.
2. Bazzi P, Moggio M, Prelle A, et al. Critically ill patients: immunological evidence of inflammation in muscle biopsy. *Clin Neuropathol* 1999;18:23–30.
3. Bindels LB, Delzenne NM. Muscle wasting: the gut microbiota as a new therapeutic target? *Int J Biochem Cell Biol* 2013;45:2186–2190.
4. Brunner R, Rinner W, Haberler C, et al. Early treatment with IgM-enriched intravenous immunoglobulin does not mitigate critical illness polyneuropathy and/or myopathy in patients with multiple organ failure and SIRS/sepsis: a prospective, randomized, placebo-controlled, double-blinded trial. *Crit Care* 2013;17:R213.
5. Cartwright MS, Kwayisi G, Griffin LP, et al. Quantitative neuromuscular ultrasound in the intensive care unit. *Muscle Nerve* 2013;47:255–259.
6. Chambers MA, Moylan JS, Reid MB. Physical inactivity and muscle weakness in the critically ill. *Crit Care Med* 2009;37:S337–S346.
7. de Jonghe B, Lacherade JC, Sharshar T, Outin H. Intensive care unit-acquired weakness: risk factors and prevention. *Crit Care Med* 2009;37:S309–S315.
8. Druschky A, Herkert M, Radespiel-Troger M, et al. Critical illness polyneuropathy: clinical findings and cell culture assay of neurotoxicity assessed by a prospective study. *Intensive Care Med* 2001;27:686–693.
9. Elke G, Schadler D, Engel C, et al. Current practice in nutritional support and its association with mortality in septic patients: results from a national, prospective, multicenter study. *Crit Care Med* 2008;36:1762–1767.
10. Fan E. What is stopping us from early mobility in the intensive care unit? *Crit Care Med* 2010;38:2254–2255.
11. Fenzi F, Latronico N, Refatti N, Rizzuto N. Enhanced expression of E-selectin on the vascular endothelium of peripheral nerve in critically ill patients with neuromuscular disorders. *Acta Neuropathol* 2003;106:75–82.
12. Gertken JT, Patel AT, Boon AJ. Electromyography and anticoagulation. *PMR* 2013;5 (5 Suppl):S3–79.
13. Grimm A, Teschner U, Porzelius C, et al. Muscle ultrasound for early assessment of critical illness neuromyopathy in severe sepsis. *Crit Care* 2013;17:R227.
14. Gruther W, Benesch T, Zorn C, et al. Muscle wasting in intensive care patients: ultrasound observation of the M. quadriceps femoris muscle layer. *J Rehabil Med* 2008;40:185–189.
15. Hanekom S, Gosselink R, Dean E, et al. The development of a clinical management algorithm for early physical activity and mobilization of critically ill patients: synthesis of evidence and expert opinion and its translation into practice. *Clin Rehabil* 2011;25:771–787.
16. Hermans G, Clerckx B, Vanhullebusch T, et al. Interobserver agreement of Medical Research Council sum-score and handgrip strength in the intensive care unit. *Muscle Nerve* 2012;45:18–25.
17. Hermans G, Van Mechelen H, Clerckx B, et al. Acute outcomes and 1-year mortality of ICU-acquired weakness: a cohort study and propensity matched analysis. *Am J Respir Crit Care Med* 2014;190:410–420.
18. Herridge MS, Batt J, Santos CD. ICU-acquired weakness, morbidity, and death. *Am J Respir Crit Care Med* 2014;190:360–362.
19. Herridge MS, Tansey CM, Matte A, et al. Functional disability 5 years after acute respiratory distress syndrome. *N Engl J Med* 2011;364:1293–1304.
20. Iwashyna TJ, Ely EW, Smith DM, Langa KM. Long-term cognitive impairment and functional disability among survivors of severe sepsis. *JAMA* 2010;304:1787–1794.
21. Khan J, Harrison TB, Rich MM, Moss M. Early development of critical illness myopathy and neuropathy in patients with severe sepsis. *Neurology* 2006;67:1421–1425.

22. Koch S, Spuler S, Deja M, et al. Critical illness myopathy is frequent: accompanying neuropathy protracts ICU discharge. *J Neurol Neurosurg Psychiatry* 2011;82:287–293.
23. Kortebein P, Ferrando A, Lombeida J, Wolfe R, Evans WJ. Effect of 10 days of bed rest on skeletal muscle in healthy older adults. *JAMA* 2007;297:1772–1774.
24. Koshy K, Zochodne DW. Neuromuscular complications of critical illness. In: Said G, Krarup C, eds. *Handbook of Clinical Neurology Series: Peripheral Nerve Disorders*. Amsterdam: Elsevier Science, 2013:759–780.
25. Kress JP, Hall JB. ICU-acquired weakness and recovery from critical illness. *N Engl J Med* 2014;370:1626–1635.
26. Lacomis D. Electrophysiology of neuromuscular disorders in critical illness. *Muscle Nerve* 2013;47:452–463.
27. Latronico N, Bertolini G, Guarneri B, et al. Simplified electrophysiological evaluation of peripheral nerves in critically ill patients: the Italian multi-centre CRIMYNE study. *Crit Care* 2007;11:R11.
28. Latronico N, Bolton CF. Critical illness polyneuropathy and myopathy: a major cause of muscle weakness and paralysis. *Lancet Neurol* 2011;10:931–941.
29. Latronico N, Tomelleri G, Filosto M. Critical illness myopathy. *Curr Opin Rheumatol* 2012;24:616–622.
30. Leijten FS, De Weerd AW, Poortvliet DC, et al. Critical illness polyneuropathy in multiple organ dysfunction syndrome and weaning from the ventilator. *Intensive Care Med* 1996;22:856–861.
31. Levine S, Biswas C, Dierov J, et al. Increased proteolysis, myosin depletion, and atrophic AKT-FOXO signaling in human diaphragm disuse. *Am J Respir Crit Care Med* 2011;183:483–490.
32. Levine S, Nguyen T, Taylor N, et al. Rapid disuse atrophy of diaphragm fibers in mechanically ventilated humans. *N Engl J Med* 2008;358:1327–1335.
33. Lipshutz AK, Gropper MA. Acquired neuromuscular weakness and early mobilization in the intensive care unit. *Anesthesiology* 2013;118:202–215.
34. Macht M, Wimbish T, Bodine C, Moss M. ICU-acquired swallowing disorders. *Crit Care Med* 2013;41:2396–2405.
35. Maramattom BV, Wijdicks EF. Acute neuromuscular weakness in the intensive care unit. *Crit Care Med* 2006;34:2835–2841.
36. Mehrholz J, Pohl M, Kugler J, Burridge J, Mückel S, Elsner B. Physical rehabilitation for critical illness myopathy and neuropathy. *Cochrane Database Syst Rev* 2015;3:CD010942.
37. Moss M, Yang M, Macht M, et al. Screening for critical illness polyneuromyopathy with single nerve conduction studies. *Intensive Care Med* 2014;40:683–690.
38. Needham DM. Mobilizing patients in the intensive care unit: improving neuromuscular weakness and physical function. *JAMA* 2008;300:1685–1690.
39. Op de Coul AA, Verheul GA, Leyten AC, Schellens RL, Teepen JL. Critical illness polyneuromyopathy after artificial respiration. *Clin Neurol Neurosurg* 1991;93:27–33.
40. Pohlman MC, Schweickert WD, Pohlman AS, et al. Feasibility of physical and occupational therapy beginning from initiation of mechanical ventilation. *Crit Care Med* 2010;38:2089–2094.
41. Puthucheary Z, Harridge S, Hart N. Skeletal muscle dysfunction in critical care: wasting, weakness, and rehabilitation strategies. *Crit Care Med* 2010;38:S676–S682.
42. Rich MM, Teener JW, Raps EC, Schotland DL, Bird SJ. Muscle is electrically inexcitable in acute quadriplegic myopathy. *Neurology* 1996;46:731–736.
43. Roberts BM, Ahn B, Smuder AJ, et al. Diaphragm and ventilatory dysfunction during cancer cachexia. *FASEB J* 2013;27:2600–2610.
44. Roubenoff R. Molecular basis of inflammation: relationships between catabolic cytokines, hormones, energy balance, and muscle. *JPEN J Parenter Enteral Nutr* 2008;32:630–632.
45. Stevens RD, Dowdy DW, Michaels RK, et al. Neuromuscular dysfunction acquired in critical illness: a systematic review. *Intensive Care Med* 2007;33:1876–1891.

46. Tzanis G, Vasileiadis I, Zervakis D, et al. Maximum inspiratory pressure, a surrogate parameter for the assessment of ICU-acquired weakness. *BMC Anesthesiol* 2011;11:14.
47. Wijdicks EFM, Fulgham JR. Failure of high dose intravenous immunoglobulins to alter the clinical course of critical illness polyneuropathy. *Muscle Nerve* 1994;17:1494–1495.
48. Wijdicks EFM. *Neurologic Complications of Critical Illness*. 3rd ed. Oxford: Oxford University Press, 2011.
49. Witteveen E, Wieske L, Verhamme C, et al. Muscle and nerve inflammation in intensive care unit-acquired weakness: a systematic translational review. *J Neurol Sci* 2014;345:15–25.
50. Zink W, Kollmar R, Schwab S. Critical illness polyneuropathy and myopathy in the intensive care unit. *Nat Rev Neurol* 2009;5:372–379.

8

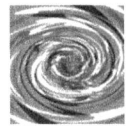

Neurology of Polytrauma

Polytrauma, it is said, changes the situation of a stable severely injured patient to that of a patient prone to rapid demise. At various defining clinical points, the management of a polytraumatized patient is in the hands of trauma surgeons, spine surgeons, and neurosurgeons.[11] Already in the emergency department, a patient's neurologic presentation may have been overshadowed by marked hypotension, blood loss, and multiple fractures needing immediate triage to the operating room. Even the neurosurgeon examining for possible traumatic brain injury (TBI) may see the patient only after an exploratory laparotomy. Jostling priorities is a common clinical stressor with surgeons and emergency physicians.

Management is ideally a multidisciplinary interplay between neurointensivists and trauma surgeons or neurosurgeons, but trauma surgeons may go at it alone. When patients are admitted to trauma units, neurologists are seldom consulted. If they are, at a certain point, specific issues are raised that can have profound implications.

Judging the severity of TBI is a common request and obviously the most pertinent one. The types of TBI are described in another volume of this series, *Handling Difficult Situations*. The initial triage of TBI is described in *Identifying Neuroemergencies* and assessment of outcome of TBI is found in *Communicating Prognosis*. A neurosurgeon consult is required for any patient with an abnormality on computed tomography (CT) scanning, but also for any patient with a major TBI. These are typically patients who have experienced a motor vehicle accident, fall, or assault and certainly includes those with open skull wounds or penetrating injury. A neurosurgeon also needs to be consulted if there is potential evidence of spinal cord injury.

New evidence of neurologic symptomatology may prompt a consultation with the neurologist. There are several important neurologic manifestations in a polytrauma patient who has injured several vital structures and organs. In many practices, the direct questions for the neurologist in specialized trauma units concentrate on five problems: What has caused sudden neurologic deterioration? Why is there new-onset or persistent coma? How can we evaluate the presentation of a new ischemic stroke and its association with blunt vascular injury? How can we recognize and rapidly manage fat embolization syndrome? What are the major peripheral nerve injuries to consider? These topics are addressed in this chapter, along with options for management.

Principles

The first core principle is that any patient with TBI is unstable during the first 48 hours—the "stable until they are not stable" phase. Attention to situations that may rapidly or suddenly change is mandated, but a patient's condition also can deteriorate due to expanding new epidural or subdural hematoma or new contusions. These conditions can cause rapidly developing fullness in the supratentorial space and increased intracranial pressure. The lesions that indicate contused brain are found on CT and can be grossly divided into diffuse axonal injury with edema, intracerebral hematoma, and combinations. In comatose patients, CT scans need to be assessed for mass effect, which can be a reason for early evacuation of the hemorrhagic contusion or placement of an intracranial pressure (ICP) monitor. The signs are displacement of the septum pellucidum or pineal gland (>1 cm), unilateral widening of the prepontine or perimesencephalic cistern caused by horizontal displacement or rotation of the brainstem, and development of obstructive hydrocephalus.

In 50% of patients with clinically certain TBI (i.e., patients who briefly lost consciousness and arrived awake but with retrograde and antegrade amnesia), the CT scan is initially normal. It is in those patients that later problems can arise. Most concerning are traumatic intracerebral hemorrhages, which often occur within hours after presentation but may be delayed (defined as >24 hours) in about half of the patients. Elderly patients in their 70s–80s are predominantly at risk for such a clinical course. The initial CT scan will show some mild subarachnoid hemorrhage, but then hematoma form from expanding and blossoming contusions in the frontal and temporal lobes. Some of these patients may acutely deteriorate with a need for intubation and may even develop an acute fixed dilated pupil if there is a temporal lobe blowout.

The most dangerous locations are in the posterior fossa. A traumatic hematoma may suddenly cause a clinical deterioration, most often in children. These hemorrhages originate from the transverse sinus and are immediately life-threatening because of the small compartment under the tentorium. Very little additional volume is needed to fill this space and cause denting of the brainstem or obliteration of the fourth ventricle, leading to obstructive hydrocephalus.

Acute diffuse brain swelling within 24 hours after admission results from a severe axonal injury and is typically seen in patients who are stuporous, comatose, and intubated after a traumatic head injury. A repeat CT scan will show diffuse severe edema that is quite apparent and with multilocalized white-matter shears.

Any assessment of TBI by a physician requires a detailed description of the CT scan findings. Marshall's classification is most often used in prognostic models but is not so common in clinical practice, and such sufficient detailed documentation is rarely found (Table 8.1).[20] However, the classification was originally devised not only to help one prognosticate and assess severity but also to help find patients who are at high risk for increased ICP and to determine a need to have an ICP monitor placed. Indirectly, this would indicate some measure of severity, but "bad-looking" CT scans do not always coincide with "bad-looking" patients—some have a normal ICP. As with any scale or score, however, it assists the attending physicians to look at the CT scan more systematically and allows them to be more concise and accurate in their communication. Grade

Table 8.1 **Marshall's Computed Tomography (CT) Classification of Diffuse Brain Injury**

Category	Definition
I	No visible intracranial disease on CT scan
II	Cisterns present
	Midline shift of 0–5 mm or lesion density or both
	No high- or mixed-density lesion >25 mL
	May include bone fragments and foreign bodies
III	Cisterns compressed or absent
	Midline shift of 0–5 mm
	No high- or mixed-density lesion >25 mL
IV	Midline shift >5 mm
	No high- or mixed-density lesion >25 mL

From Marshall et al.[20]

III or IV diffuse axonal injury has the best correlation with ICP, justifying aggressive management and monitoring of ICP (and other parameters if available). Otherwise, the scale is not a detailed CT classification of TBI and better scales are unquestionably needed. Nonetheless, if abnormalities are seen on the CT scan that could potentially indicate increased ICP, one should immediately elevate the head of the bed 30 degrees and treat with hyperosmotic solutions such as 20% mannitol (1 g/kg) or hypertonic saline (3% NaCl 150 mL IV over 10 minutes). Clinical judgment combined with CT scan readings may justify such an approach, and later treatment can be guided by ICP monitoring.

The role of the consulting neurologist may thus be quite important, helping to determine whether ICP monitoring is warranted and when it is needed urgently. Neurologists may also call for a neurosurgeon if this has not already been done, in particular if there is a contusion with mass effect. Our experience in patients seen in trauma ICU has been just that—to treat ICP when needed and to guide to more multidisciplinary involvement. Further practical advice on TBI recognition and management can be found in the volume *Handling Difficult Situations*.

The second core principle is that the neurologist is also often asked to evaluate spinal cord injury. Fractures and dislocations of the spine are likely to have contused the spinal cord. However, hyperextension strain is known to exhibit very few radiologic features. Some prevertebral swelling or avulsion fractures may be seen in a patient with a complete spinal cord lesion. More conspicuous lesions associated with spinal cord injury are traumatic spondylolisthesis of the second cervical vertebra (C2), known as a hangman's fracture; burst fracture of the cervical body with disk material and bone fragments forced into the spinal canal; and bilateral cervical facet dislocation. Similarly, fracture dislocation in the thoracic area increases the likelihood of spinal cord injury.

It is key that spinal cord injury is recognized immediately. Comatose patients with TBI may have no motor response, hypotension, or bradycardia due to increased vagal function not corrected by lost sympathetic neuronal input, and each of these signs may be inaccurately attributed to hypovolemic shock. Unrecognized urinary retention may occur because of an atonic bladder. Often, the patient's breathing seems markedly labored early; a relatively normal chest radiograph may provide a clue that respiratory mechanics are at fault. Some patients were intubated in the field, making it even more difficult to recognize apnea caused by cervical cord injury.

Spinal cord examination requires—at the very least—determination of a sensory level (e.g., nipple T4, navel T10) and testing of key muscles going down the segments step by step: deltoid and biceps C5, brachioradialis C6, triceps C7, wrist flexors C8, interossei T1, quadriceps L3, tibialis anterior L4, extensor hallucis longus L5, and gastrocnemius S1. Using these muscles and the sensory level, an approximate lesion can be deduced. The American Spinal Injury Association scale can be used to determine whether the lesion is complete (A) or incomplete (B/C, where B represents preserved sensory function and C represents preserved motor function below the level of injury). Management of acute spinal cord injury is discussed in more detail in the volume *Handling Difficult Situations*.

The third core principle is to recognize an acute ischemic stroke after blunt vascular trauma (Figure 8.1).[1,15,24] This may occur as a result of cervical spine injury, and it can involve both acute carotid artery and vertebral artery dissections. These traumatic dissections are often underdiagnosed. A computed tomography angiogram (CTA)

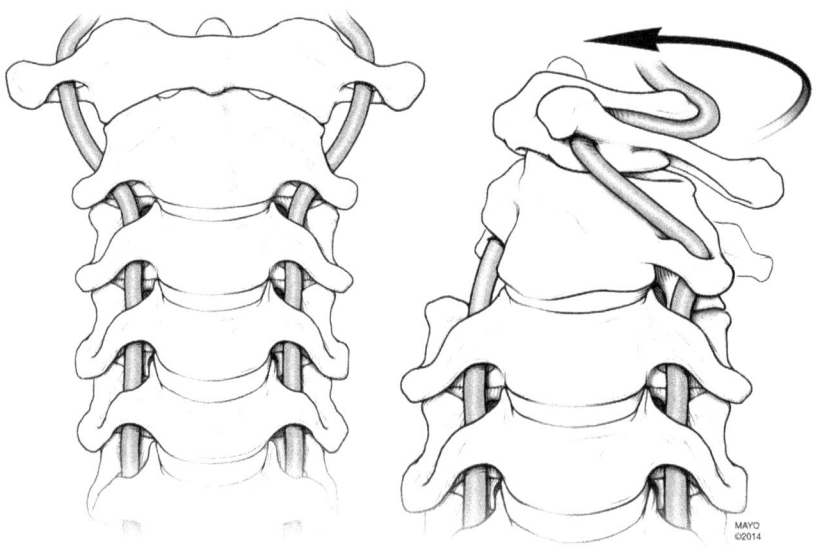

Figure 8.1 Mechanism of traumatic vertebral artery injury as a result of forceful rotation.

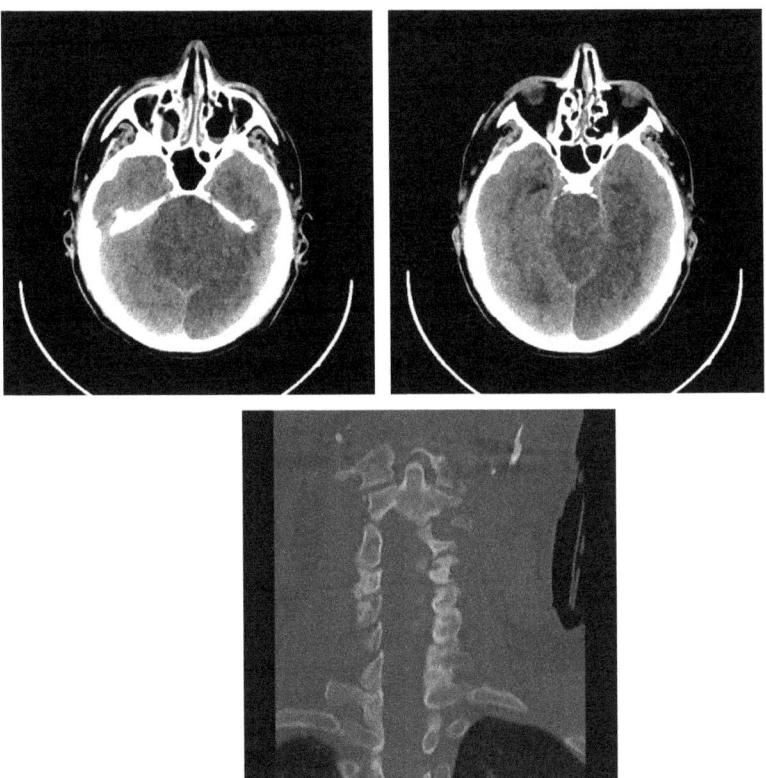

Figure 8.2 CT images show cerebral infarct in the posterior circulation after a motor vehicle accident and persistent coma. The cervical spine shows an C1 arch fracture causing vertebral dissection

is necessary to document the traumatic dissection. The prevalence might be significantly higher now with the availability of detailed CTA reconstructions.[9,10] Usually, the rapid acceleration–deceleration injury stretches arteries, resulting primarily in an intimal tear, which leads to luminal narrowing and eventually to occlusion and injury. Ischemic injury can come from immediate occlusion of the artery and may explain a large territorial infarction in a patient with TBI (Figure 8.2). Smaller watershed infarcts can be seen. Symptoms occur more than 12 hours after impact, and this delayed course has been reported in 25%–50% of patients. Later embolization—up to 1 week—has also been recorded. Generally, carotid and vertebral dissections cause infarcts in cerebral and cerebellar hemispheres, but vertebral artery dissection may cause both cervical spine and medulla oblongata infarctions. Three-dimensional CT is often able to document the presence of a traumatic aneurysm that will further complicate management.

There are several physical findings that can predict high risk of injury to cerebrovascular arteries; they are shown in Table 8.2. Both the Denver and the Memphis criteria (Table 8.3) point toward these injuries. Other findings that increase the risk

Table 8.2 **Factors and Physical Findings Associated with Blunt Trauma of Cerebral Vasculature after TBI**

Cervical bruit
Cervical hematoma
Cervical spine injury
Cranial nerve injury
Facial and skull fractures
Horner's syndrome
Intraoral trauma
Neck soft-tissue injury
Oropharyngeal, nasal, or auricular hemorrhage
Pulsatile tinnitus
Seatbelt sign
Spinal cord injury
Thoracic trauma

are the seatbelt sign, the occurrence of cranial fractures, and evidence of a direct blow to the head resulting in facial fractures.

The fourth core principle is to recognize that a secondary deterioration in a patient with polytrauma can result from sudden mobilization of multiple fat particles. Fat embolization syndrome is typically seen in patients who have a long-bone fracture (e.g., humerus, femur).[4,14,17,21,22] It may be seen after initial stabilization and pinning of the fracture suggesting manipulation may have provoked it. The clinical criteria for fat embolization include new development of tachypnea, tachycardia, sudden hypoxemia,

Table 8.3 **Screening Protocols for Blunt Trauma of Cerebral Vasculature**

Denver criteria	Memphis criteria
Any cervical spine fracture	Cervical spine fracture
Unexplained neurologic deficit	Neurological deficit not explained by brain imaging
Basilar cranial fracture into carotid canal	Basilar cranial fracture into carotid canal
Le Fort II or III fracture	Le Fort II or III fracture
Cervical hematoma	Horner's syndrome
Cervical bruit	Neck soft-tissue injury
Ischemic stroke	
Coma and Head injury	
Hanging with anoxic injury	

Adapted From Fusco and Harrigan.[10]

sudden intubation and requirement for high positive end-expiratory pressure (PEEP), and in acute respiratory distress syndrome. However, pulmonary findings may be subtle or not clearly present. Patients may, within an hour, lapse into coma showing worrisome extensor posturing.

Fat embolization from bone marrow of recently fractured long bones occurs most often in patients with multitrauma. In general, within 12–24 hours after the initial traumatic impact, the patient's condition deteriorates. Fat embolization requires sufficient pressurization to force fat globules upward through the venous system.[16] Fat occludes multiple brain arterioles, and this is what is seen on magnetic resonance imaging (MRI)—the so-called "starfield pattern."[7,8,23,27] Sudden tachypnea and tachycardia and the development of a large alveolar–arterial oxygen gradient may be seen, with clinical indicators of the lodging of fat globules in the pulmonary vasculature. A pathognomonic sign, present in 50% of patients, is a petechial rash that appears suddenly on the chest, axillary folds, and, occasionally, conjunctiva. Many patients become "confused," and focal signs and generalized tonic–clonic seizures may occur. The clinical diagnosis becomes fairly certain when at least one major and four minor criteria are present (Table 8.4). In patients without pulmonary symptoms, cerebral fat embolization can at times be explained by a patent foramen ovale. In others, the pathway of fat globules—small enough to pass through the lungs—is presumably similar to that of air emboli.

The fifth core principle is to consider traumatic aneurysms when there are frontal lobe hemorrhages located close to a falx or interhemispheric fissure.[6,25,29] Traumatic intracranial aneurysms are rare, but usually occur in the anterior cerebral artery. They are typically saccular, but not at branching points. This location is explained by rubbing of the cerebral artery against the falx. Cranial fractures are present in approximately 90% of patients with traumatic intracranial aneurysms. Intracranial aneurysms can rupture and approximately 50% of them within the first week after they have been found. Aggressive treatment is necessary. Endovascular treatment is rarely performed (7% of cases in a National Trauma Database Study).[19]

The sixth core principle to remember is that the presence of a monoplegia can be related to an isolated neuropathy associated with fracture. Isolated nerve injuries and plexopathies are uncommon in patients with multitrauma and require the expertise of neurosurgeons and orthopedic surgeons. The three major arm nerves can be injured by a bone fracture, but usually only one nerve is involved. Fractures of the ulna have been associated with complete paralysis of the anterior interosseous nerve, a motor branch of the median nerve. A characteristic feature is weakness of the flexor

Table 8.4 **Gurd's Criteria for Fat Embolization Syndrome**

Major feature	Minor feature	Laboratory findings
Petechial rash	Pyrexia	Anemia
Respiratory failure	Tachycardia	Thrombocytopenia
Neurologic involvement	Retinal changes	Elevated erythrocyte sedimentation rate
	Jaundice	Fat macroglobulinemia
	Renal failure	

pollicis longus or flexor digitorum profundus and pronator quadratus without any sensory deficit. Patients may notice abnormal pinching, which can easily be demonstrated when they are asked to make a circle with the thumb and index finger. Acute median nerve damage is associated with wrist fractures. Entrapment of the ulnar nerve at the elbow region may occur in supracondylar humeral fractures. Neurolysis with anterior transposition has resulted in satisfactory outcomes. The most common lesion is radial nerve paralysis associated with fractures of the humerus. Fortunately, clinical recovery is expected within 1 month in one third of these patients, and the remainder improves within 6 months. Other peripheral nerve injuries are axillary nerve damage (from anterior dislocation of the shoulder) and damage to the sciatic nerve (from dislocation of the acetabulum of the pelvis), both with potential for complete recovery.

A proximal brachial plexopathy is associated with Horner's syndrome and may also be associated with unilateral paralysis of the diaphragm. Most of the time, these injuries produce complete paralysis of all arm musculature, resulting in a flaccid, immobile, and hypostatic limb.

Traumatic brachial plexus palsy is frequently seen in young patients after motorcycle accidents.[2,13,18,26] In the initial assessment of brachial plexus injuries, careful evaluation of the magnitude of nerve damage is important, because later secondary deterioration may be associated with the development of a false aneurysm or an arteriovenous fistula in an axillary artery, requiring immediate surgical intervention.

Closed brachial plexus injuries may be approached by differentiating patients who have a proximal injury from those who have a postganglionic injury. Proximal brachial plexus injury is manifested by Horner's syndrome (C8 to T1), winging of the scapula, and paralysis of the rhomboids. Diaphragmatic paralysis is occasionally present.[18] Electromyographic and sensory nerve studies are usually performed 6–8 weeks after the initial insult and may differentiate a preganglionic from a postganglionic lesion. Normal sensory conduction from the anesthetic median or radial nerve area of the hand strongly suggests a preganglionic injury at the C6–C7 level. Somatosensory studies may also be helpful. Subsequently, CT myelography or MRI is done to exclude rootlet avulsion in case plexus repair is considered. (For most patients, 3 months must have elapsed without spontaneous improvement.[28])

Similarly, in postganglionic injuries of the brachial plexus, operative repair is considered if no clinical or electromyographic improvement is found after 3 months. Detailed discussion of nerve repair techniques can be found in textbooks and review articles. Nerve root avulsion of the brachial plexus is the most devastating injury, but palliative therapy and control of pain, which can be excruciating for some patients, is possible. Complete paralysis or some remaining flicker of movement in the deltoid, supraspinous, or biceps muscle may be found, and all sensation is lost. A recent provocative study of 10 patients examined the effects of reimplantation of avulsed ventral roots through slits in the pia mater and spinal cord surface. Three of the patients had a small degree of recovery, with resistance in some muscles and biceps strength to overcome gravity. Joint position improved in some, and pain was reduced.

Injury to the lumbosacral plexus, which is far less common than traumatic brachial plexus injury, can result from compression or stretching of the plexus in sacral and pelvic fractures. External iliac artery injury occasionally accompanies the nerve damage. An MRI study may be useful in establishing lumbosacral nerve root avulsion, which precludes operative correction. The outcome of traumatic lumbosacral plexus injury is unpredictable and often poor.

In Practice

It is difficult to carefully neurologically examine a patient who has just survived a major multisystem or crush trauma. Many patients are treated with high doses of fentanyl and some patients are casted or in traction. Some patients require neuromuscular junction blockers to better manage mechanical ventilation for pulmonary injury. CT scans are difficult to obtain considering the risks of transport. There is understandable reluctance to evaluate a patient with so many confounders and with so many restrictions.

Much of the management in a polytrauma patient focuses on management of traumatic head injury and often includes placement of an ICP monitor (and brain oxygen monitor in specialized TBI centers). Placement of a parenchymal monitoring device is needed for any patient with a motor response that is less than localizing and a CT scan showing absence of basal cisterns, intraventricular or subarachnoid blood, or an intracerebral contusion. It is even more imperative if sedation or neuromuscular junction blockers are needed to manage a flail chest. Current recommendations call for immediate reduction of ICP to less than 20 mm Hg and maintenance of cerebral perfusion pressure at greater than 60 mm Hg. PEEP mode is often necessary to ensure adequate oxygenation in patients with additional lung trauma. Decreased lung compliance in those patients with acute lung concussion or flail chest most likely prevents transmural conductance of airway pressure to the right atrium and eventually to the cerebral venous system, and thus PEEP rarely raises ICP.

If there is no consistent response to treatment with the maximal dose of mannitol (2 g/kg) and no evidence of a new neurosurgical lesion (e.g., an epidural or subdural hematoma), a more aggressive treatment is used. Hypertonic saline (23%, 30–60 mL in 15 minutes) may be added and will have a more profound effect. Repeated doses may be needed, aiming at a serum sodium level of 150 mmol/L. (The chloride portion in hypertonic saline can cause a severe metabolic acidosis—it can easily be replaced with acetate by the ICU pharmacist.) Refractory intracranial hypertension may warrant hemi- or bifrontal craniectomy. This procedure often controls ICP.

Patients with an acute subdural hematoma due to ruptured bridging veins typically may become drowsy or comatose at presentation. In many patients, an associated cerebral contusion is found, and outcome is presumably related to diffuse TBI rather than to the effect of brain shift alone. Acute subdural hematoma remains associated with high mortality in the elderly and old age (defined as >65 years) and quadruples the mortality rate. However, prognostication in the early postoperative weeks remains unreliable and patient may improve substantially. Improvement is more likely if seizures are detected on continuous EEG monitoring and these generalized periodic epileptic discharges are appropriately treated.

If patients decline rapidly, frontal and temporal contusional hematomas will likely be removed by a neurosurgeon, and additional partial lobe resection maybe be performed if the location is in the nondominant hemisphere. Hematomas in the deep white matter are treated medically in many large trauma centers.

The treatment of traumatic injury to cerebral vessels is unknown, but most patients are given a short course of dual antiplatelet therapy.[3] This treatment will only partly prevent later embolization. Use of intravenous heparin has been associated with an increased hemorrhagic complication rate, particularly in the setting of polytrauma. Most centers prefer aspirin and clopidogrel rather than intravenous heparin. Endovascular treatment is eventually necessary if there is an expanding traumatic aneurysm; this may involve stenting with balloon-expandable stents or embolization of the aneurysm with coils.[5,12]

The next questions to ask are whether the current level of consciousness can be adequately explained and whether more structural injuries might be expected. Imaging plays a major role, including CTA of great vessels (carotid, vertebral, aortic arch). CT can provide evidence of ischemic strokes in the posterior circulation, in particular because the vertebral arteries are vulnerable to trauma.

Fat embolization syndrome remains difficult to prove. The CT scan of the brain is often normal, but MRI is diagnostic (Figure 8.3). There is no proven treatment, and management is largely supportive, often with mechanical ventilation until the patient's level of consciousness improves. Corticosteroids have no role in the treatment of fat embolization syndrome. Fat embolism syndrome can be rapidly fatal, but in most patients, clinical signs resolve within 24 hours, and the outcome can be surprisingly good.[23] Prognosis has been good in approximately two thirds of the reported cases, but improvement can be gradual, so de-escalation of care would be premature

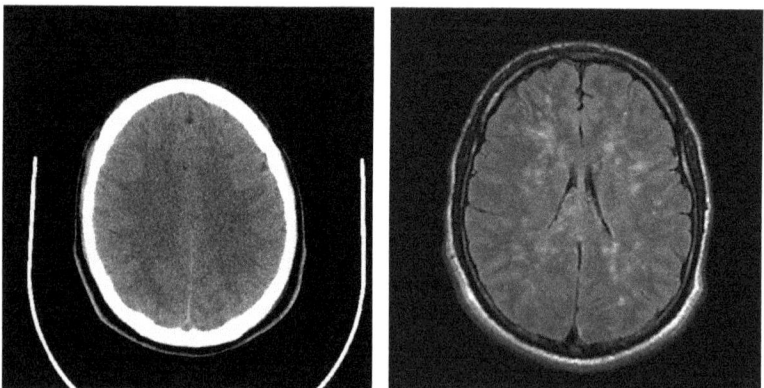

Figure 8.3 In this example of cerebral fat embolization, the CT was considered normal, but there were tiny hypodense specks in the white matter that could represent fat. On MRI, a starfield pattern was shown using fluid attenuation inversion recovery sequence.

and frankly inappropriate. Treatment should be focused on immediate stabilization of the fracture.

The spinal cord and brachial plexus may be simultaneously injured in about 10% of patients with polytrauma.[18] The presence of associated injuries (e.g., cervical fractures, supraclavicular vascular injuries) and preganglionic injury signs and symptoms (e.g., Horner's syndrome, preoperative pain, phrenic nerve dysfunction, pseudomeningoceles) increases the probability of an associated spinal cord injury. This recognition is important, because poor surgical outcomes have been reported in patients with spinal cord injury and a concomitant brachial plexus injury. Some have argued that the spasticity associated with the upper motor neuron lesion could result in compromised sensorimotor function.[19] Whatever the explanation, brachial plexus injury is best further investigated by electromyographic and sensory nerve studies performed 6–8 weeks after the accident, as described earlier in this chapter. Close involvement of neurosurgeons is needed in any of these serious cases.

Putting It All Together

- TBI may be associated with delayed presentation of hematomas.
- Consider ICP monitoring in comatose patients with TBI and certain CT patterns.
- Arterial injury to extracerebral vessels is more common with severe polytrauma or crush injury.
- Fat embolism is rarely diagnosed and is subtle in presentation.
- Brachial plexus lesions and spinal cord lesions may coexist.
- Mononeuropathies are associated with certain fractures.

By the Way

- Hypotension may occur with acute spinal cord injury.
- Severe hypotension can cause ischemic optic neuropathy and blindness.
- Crush injury involves arterial dissection and may cause cerebral infarctions.
- Cardiac arrest after polytrauma may have caused anoxic-ischemic brain injury.

Neurology of Polytrauma by the Numbers

- ~60% of severe TBI is part of serious polytrauma.
- ~50% of delayed traumatic hematomas occur after 24 hours.
- ~30% of delayed traumatic hematomas require urgent surgery.
- ~25% of carotid blunt injuries involve a luminal irregularity.
- ~25% of severe TBI is associated with spinal cord injury.

References

1. Arthurs ZM, Starnes BW. Blunt carotid and vertebral artery injuries. *Injury* 2008; 39:1232–1241.
2. Bekelis K, Missios S, Spinner RJ. Restraints and peripheral nerve injuries in adult victims of motor vehicle crashes. *J Neurotrauma* 2014;31:1077–1082.
3. Blacker DJ, Wijdicks EF. Clinical characteristics and mechanisms of stroke after polytrauma. *Mayo Clin Proc* 2004;79:630–635.
4. Bulger EM, Smith DG, Maier RV, Jurkovich GJ. Fat embolism syndrome: a 10-year review. *Arch Surg* 1997;132:435–439.
5. Chaer RA, Derubertis B, Kent KC, McKinsey JF. Endovascular treatment of traumatic carotid pseudoaneurysm with stenting and coil embolization. *Ann Vasc Surg* 2008;22:564–567.
6. Chen D, Concus AP, Halbach VV, Cheung SW. Epistaxis originating from traumatic pseudoaneurysm of the internal carotid artery: diagnosis and endovascular therapy. *Laryngoscope* 1998;108:326–331.
7. Chen JJ, Ha JC, Mirvis SE. MR imaging of the brain in fat embolism syndrome. *Emerg Radiol* 2008;15:187–192.
8. Citerio G, Bianchini E, Beretta L. Magnetic resonance imaging of cerebral fat embolism: a case report. *Intensive Care Med* 1995;21:679–681.
9. Fusco MR, Harrigan MR. Cerebrovascular dissections: a review. Part I: spontaneous dissections. *Neurosurgery* 2011;68:242–257.
10. Fusco MR, Harrigan MR. Cerebrovascular dissections: a review. Part II: blunt cerebrovascular injury. *Neurosurgery* 2011;68:517–530.
11. Harrois A, Hamada S, Laplace C, Duranteau J, Vigue B. The initial management of severe trauma patients at hospital admission. *Ann Fr Anesth Reanim* 2013;32:483–491.
12. Hauck EF, Natarajan SK, Horvathy DB, et al. Stent-assisted basilar reconstruction for a traumatic vertebral dissection with a large basilar artery thrombosis. *J Neurointerv Surg* 2011;3:47–49.
13. Kachramanoglou C, Li D, Andrews P, et al. Novel strategies in brachial plexus repair after traumatic avulsion. *Br J Neurosurg* 2011;25:16–27.
14. Kellogg RG, Fontes RB, Lopes DK. Massive cerebral involvement in fat embolism syndrome and intracranial pressure management. *J Neurosurg* 2013;119:1263–1270.
15. Koleilat I, Gandhi R, Boulos A, Bonville D. Traumatic bilateral carotid and vertebral artery dissection. *J Emerg Trauma Shock* 2014;7:47–48.
16. Kosova E, Bergmark B, Piazza G. Fat embolism syndrome. *Circulation* 2015;13:317–320.
17. Levy D. The fat embolism syndrome: a review. *Clin Orthop Relat Res* 1990;261:281–286.
18. Limthongthang R, Bachoura A, Songcharoen P, Osterman AL. Adult brachial plexus injury: evaluation and management. *Orthop Clin North Am* 2013;44:591–603.
19. Majidi S, Hassan AE, Adil MM, Jadhav V, Qureshi AI. Incidence and outcome of vertebral artery dissection in trauma setting: analysis of national trauma data base. *Neurocritical Care* 2014;21:253–258.
20. Marshall LF, Eisenberg H, Jane JA, Marshall SB, Klauber MR. A new classification of head injury based on computerized tomography. *J Neurosurg* 1991;75:S14-S20.
21. Mellor A, Soni N. Fat embolism. *Anaesthesia* 2001;56:145–154.
22. Metting Z, Rodiger LA, Regtien JG, van der Naalt J. Delayed coma in head injury: consider cerebral fat embolism. *Clin Neurol Neurosurg* 2009;111:597–600.
23. Mittal MK, Burrus TM, Campeau NG, et al. Pearls & oy-sters: good recovery following cerebral fat embolization with paroxysmal hyperactivity syndrome. *Neurology* 2013; 81:e107–e109.
24. Mortazavi MM, Verma K, Tubbs RS, Harrigan M. Pediatric traumatic carotid, vertebral and cerebral artery dissections: a review. *Childs Nerv Syst* 2011;27:2045–2056.
25. Nakstad P, Nornes H, Hauge HN. Traumatic aneurysms of the pericallosal arteries. *Neuroradiology* 1986;28:335–338.

26. O'Shea K, Feinberg JH, Wolfe SW. Imaging and electrodiagnostic work-up of acute adult brachial plexus injuries. *J Hand Surg Eur Vol* 2011;36:747–759.
27. Pfeffer G, Heran MK. Restricted diffusion and poor clinical outcome in cerebral fat embolism syndrome. *Can J Neurol Sci* 2010;37:128–130.
28. Tagliafico A, Altafini L, Garello I, et al. Traumatic neuropathies: spectrum of imaging findings and postoperative assessment. *Semin Musculoskelet Radiol* 2010;14:512–522.
29. Yang TC, Lo YL, Huang YC, Yang ST. Traumatic anterior cerebral artery aneurysm following blunt craniofacial trauma. *Eur Neurol* 2007;58:239–245.

9

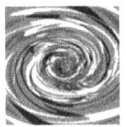

Neurooncologic Emergencies

Patients with advanced cancer are admitted to the ward for further diagnostic or surgical purposes, but they may be transferred to an intensive care unit (ICU) if a major complication occurs. Not infrequently, patients "code" or require renal replacement therapies necessitating urgent intubation and transfer. Most physicians, understandably, think that deterioration in patients with advanced cancer should be considered a questionable indication for transfer to an ICU, because these patients are perceived to have very poor outcome if sepsis intervenes or mechanical ventilation is needed.[18,31,36,38] In many clinical practices, poor performance status, presence of recurrence or rapid progression, or serious cancer-related complications may preclude transfer and more often there is an agreement to transition to palliation. Therefore, the number of ICU admissions of advanced cancer patients is low (<5%). Nonetheless, patients without a definite poor outlook may benefit from critical care—at least for a period of time.

Neurologic complications of cancer are common because cancer is common in general hospitals and also because most data are from cancer hospitals, creating a major referral bias. Neurooncology also is limited in therapeutic options, and many neurooncologists diagnose and refer patients for treatment, but then see them only after they have progressed. Neurologic disorders relate to metastases, vascular complications, side effects of radiation and chemotherapy, and paraneoplastic syndromes.

Emergencies often occur in patients admitted to ICUs. Many of these oncologic emergencies relate to new onset of neurologic symptoms or declining consciousness. Neurologic manifestations may also occur with major malignancy-induced complications such as tumor lysis syndrome and hypercalcemia, the development of acute superior vena cava syndrome or other vascular disorders, hemorrhage from abdominal cancer, electrolyte imbalance, hypoglycemia, and major systemic infections causing sepsis—some related to febrile neutropenia. Neurologists are definitively consulted when carcinomatous meningitis is considered or has been recently discovered, when patients are admitted with brain metastases on computed tomography scans, when there is an urgency with malignant spinal cord compression, and regarding any other acute manifestation of a presumed paraneoplastic syndrome. There may be an unexpected new mass lesion.

The number of neurologic complications associated with cancer is substantial, and readers are referred to major textbooks on the topic.[7,8,32] Recognition and management of paraneoplastic limbic encephalitis or autoimmune encephalitis in the setting of previously undiagnosed cancer is discussed in another volume in this series, *Handling Difficult Situations*. The most relevant questions that are often asked are the following: Does the patient need immediate intervention for brain edema associated with metastases? Does the patient need acute neurosurgical intervention for spinal cord compression? Is there evidence of acute cerebrovascular disease associated with compression of vascular structures? What immunotherapy options are to be considered in paraneoplastic syndromes? Is the neurologic manifestation part of an acute metabolic derangement? This chapter provides a discussion of the most frequent consultations for patients with advanced cancer who become critically ill and appear to have developed a neurologic sign.

Principles

The first core principle is to have a sense of the patient mix in the ICU. Over the years, the admitted population has changed and the most common reasons for these patients to be in the ICU, accounting for probably up to 80%, are common problems such as sepsis, septic shock and acute respiratory failure requiring mechanical ventilation.[1]

Many patients have hematologic malignancies, and they are particularly at risk for poor outcome when mechanical ventilation is required. ICU admission for a hematologic malignancy may also relate to hematopoietic stem cell transplantation. Mortality in this population of patients is again associated with multiorgan system failure and shock, and is still between 60% and 70% among patients with hematologic cancer.[3] Some have questioned whether patients who have recently undergone hematopoietic stem cell transplantation benefit from ICU transfer for monitoring,[20] but it is now recognized that there is a chance that outcome can be improved.

In one study on outcome in oncology ICU patients, the percentage of patients who died was 8% with no organ system involvement but 93% when more than 3 organ systems failed. Both the need for mechanical ventilation and need for dialysis increased ICU mortality by approximately 50%.[3,19] However, it is possible that the selection of patients in the ICU has changed and intensivists have become more aggressive knowing that some patients may survive with aggressive management. Patients with relapse or recurrence whose disease is unresponsive to therapy and those with successive failure of two organ systems are typically seriously re-evaluated regarding their need for ICU care. Several studies have found that ICU in-hospital mortality for medical cancer patients is twice as high as for patients without cancer, but no clear differences have been found between patients with ICU admission after surgery and nonsurgical ICU patients.[5]

Mechanical ventilation, more aggressive antibiotic management, improved blood product transfusion, lung protective strategies for acute respiratory distress

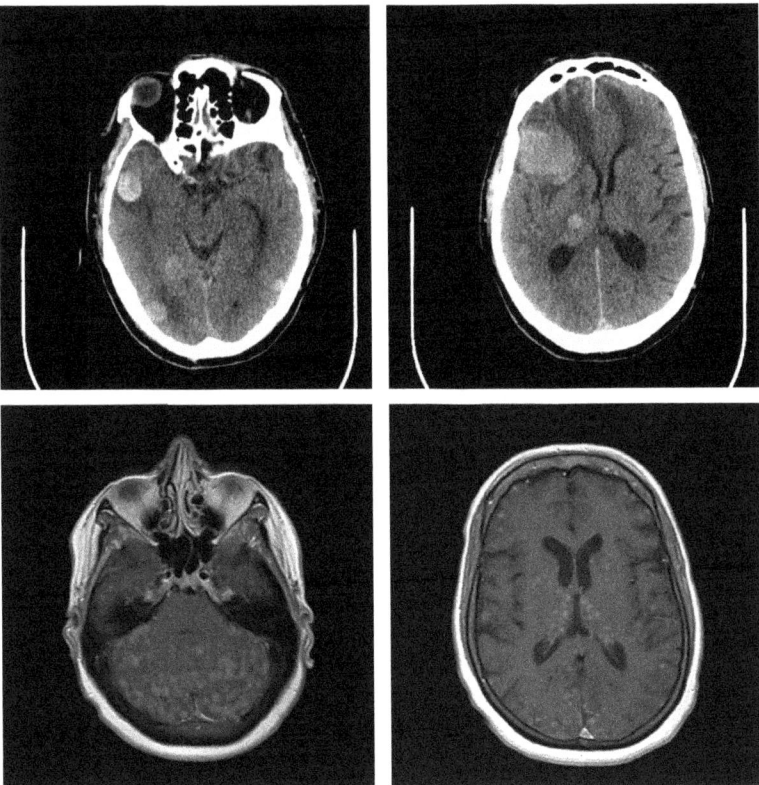

Figure 9.1 MRI reveals brain metastases: Upper row: Metastatic melanoma. Lower row: Metastatic breast cancer.

syndrome, and early intervention for severe sepsis and septic shock[38] can be all quite effective. Many patients with a solid tumor (e.g., non-Hodgkin's lymphoma, colon cancer, breast cancer) are admitted with new sepsis syndrome. Not unexpectedly, the development of multiorgan failure and need for dialysis markedly worsen the chance of a good outcome.

Thus, neurologists consulting in the ICU should expect patients with multiorgan failure or relapsed hematologic disorders, and these conditions will influence the nature of the consultation and the advice to follow. Knowing the major reasons for critical illness in cancer patients will focus the neurologist on the need for intervention.

The second core principle is that consults are usually placed because cancer has likely spread to the central nervous system (CNS) (Figure 9.1), and this can be manifested as carcinomatous meningitis or multiple brain metastases.[2,22] It may not be immediately obvious that CNS involvement is the reason for deterioration, and careful evaluation is needed. Spinal cord compression can be the first manifestation of metastasis. Any of these complications may be best imaged and defined using several

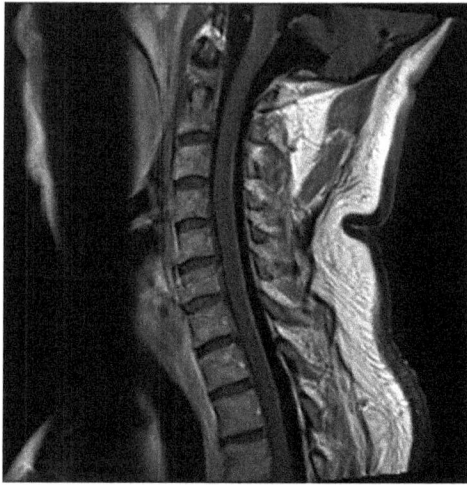

Figure 9.2 Spinal leptomeningeal carcinomatosis.

sequences on magnetic resonance imaging (MRI). Some patients require examination of the cerebrospinal fluid (CSF) to find malignant cells. MRI is highly sensitive for diagnosis of neoplastic meningitis except in patients with hematopoietic malignancies.[26] Common findings are contrast-enhanced meninges in T1-weighted sequences (Figure 9.2). If MRI is unrevealing, CSF cytology has a high sensitivity for detection of neoplastic meningitis.

A third core principle is that chemotherapy and radiation can change the neurologic picture quickly. Over time, cancer drugs produce a peripheral neuropathy. The estimates of chemotherapy-associated polyneuropathy are widely divergent, but drugs that are notorious for this side effect include bortezomib (for treatment of multiple myeloma),[17] platinum-based drugs such as cisplatinum and oxaliplatin (colon cancer), vincristine (non-Hodgkin's lymphoma), and paclitaxel (many solid tumors).[41] Many chemotherapeutic agents produce a diffuse peripheral neuropathy that may be persistent.[21] These agents initiate a "dieback" process starting from distal nerve endings as a result of impaired cytoplasmic flow. Initially, few abnormalities are found; progression occurs months after the discontinuation of treatment—a phenomenon known as "coasting." The highest risk among all platinum-based drugs is with oxaliplatin.[42,43]

Acute CNS syndromes causing acute encephalopathy and seizures have been reported with ifosfamide (for treatment of solid tumors), busulfan (hematologic cancers), and methotrexate (leukemias). Patients may develop a leukoencephalopathy, usually 24–48 hours after infusion, but mostly in exceptional severe cases. Some of the chemotherapy-associated complications are associated with posterior reversible encephalopathy syndrome. This association has been most consistently described with cyclophosphamide, sorafenib, bevacizumab, interferon alpha, and cisplatin.[16,24,37,39,40] Most oncologists have not seen a severe acute encephalopathy with chemotherapy—it is a rare and unusual complication.

The fourth core principle is to identify possible acute metabolic derangements that can produce neurologic symptoms and may have caused the critical illness. Acute tumor lysis syndrome is often associated with metabolic derangements and is a direct consequence of rapid cell lysis during treatment of hematologic malignancies.[4] These patients often have multiple myeloma, acute myeloid leukemia, or solid tumors. Tumor lysis syndrome can also occur in the setting of systemic chemotherapy or even radiation therapy. The major acute metabolic change is the presence of hyperkalemia, hyperphosphatemia, hyperuricemia, and hypocalcemia, which may produce rapidly developing encephalopathy and delirium but also significant muscle weakness and tetany. Spasms in extremities may occur; they are easily identified clinically and can be improved with calcium administration. Because renal impairment is often a rapid consequence of tumor lysis syndrome, acute uremic encephalopathy should be considered in patients with this syndrome.

Muscle cramps and paresthesias are commonly seen with hypocalcemia. Seizures may also be seen in marked hyperphosphatemia with levels greater than 1 mmol/L or a 50% increase from baseline. Hypocalcemia can result in muscle cramps and tetany, and eventually in significant cardiac arrhythmias. Malignancy-associated hypercalcemia, expected in advanced multiple myeloma and leukemias, should be immediately recognized—most of the time, it becomes apparent because of a prolonged PR interval, widening QRS complexes, and bradyarrhythmias. The clinical signs of hypercalcemia are basically dehydration and marked hypotension requiring fluid resuscitation. Some patients develop seizures, but this is unusual.

Hypoglycemia is also more commonly seen in patients with advanced cancer, particularly if there are liver metastases—it should be particularly considered in any cachectic cancer patient. Some of these hypoglycemic events are profound, with glucose levels lower than 30 mg/dL. Long-term treatment includes diazoxide, which inhibits secretion of insulin or glucagon by the pancreas.[15] Cancer-induced hypoglycemia may relate to severely reduced glucose intake or glucose synthesis. This may occur as a result of primary problems in the liver (metastasis), large tumors metabolizing large amounts of glucose, or insulin-like growth factor produced by a tumor. Fluctuations toward both marked hyperglycemia and hypoglycemia may be seen, but because of the absence of glucogenesis, hypoglycemia is more common, particularly if the patient has type 2 diabetes treated with insulin. Hyperglycemia that develops into a severe nonketotic hyperosmolar coma may be seen in patients (typically older diabetics) who have received high-dose corticosteroids—usually, in the setting of a CNS metastasis when there has been marked tissue shift from brain edema surrounding the lesion. Other electrolyte abnormalities that are less common but might be seen in any sick patient include hyponatremia and hypernatremia, but not in extreme values that could produce seizures or myoclonus or stupor.

Several paraneoplastic endocrinopathies[27] have been recognized, but most do not produce specific neurologic phenotypes. Syndrome of inappropriate antidiuretic hormone (SIADH) affects only 1% of all patients with cancer, and about half of them have small-cell lung cancer (SCLC).[33] Many chemotherapeutic agents stimulate antidiuretic hormone or worsen hyponatremia through vomiting after use of large amounts of opioids to treat pain.[29] Treatment is fluid restriction, and because serum sodium values uncommonly decrease below 125 mmol/L, hypertonic saline is not frequently used. Arginine vasopressin receptor antagonists may cause rapid correction, but the risk of osmotic demyelination and central pontine myelinolysis is not known. It would be realistic to think that malnourished, frail, and terminally ill cancer patients are at higher risk.

Cushing's syndrome due to adrenocorticotropic hormone–producing SCLC or prolonged use of high-dose corticosteroids leads to severe proximal weakness from steroid myopathy. Corticosteroids likely impair the buildup of muscle protein. The risk is very high if dexamethasone (16 mg or more daily) has been administered for 2 weeks. The proximal weakness is noted with rising from a chair or lifting objects. Muscle biopsies are rarely helpful because it will only show nonspecific type II muscle fiber loss.

In Practice

Spread of cancer to the CNS (brain and spine) may manifest with seizures, confusion and cognitive decline, headache, new deficit (hemiparesis or paraparesis), or new pain. The first course of action is to determine whether there is a structural lesion on computed tomography scan or MRI. In clinical practice, a positron emission tomography scan is additionally helpful because it can help in staging—showing the spread and the primary tumor. There is a specific approach for each of these abnormalities. The presenting symptoms are further characterized in the following sections.

PRESENTING SEMIOLOGY OF NEUROONCOLOGIC EMERGENCIES

Seizures are common at presentation in patients with metastases (20%) and also in those with neoplastic meningitis (10%). Seizures are caused by metastatic lesions that are cortically located and those that are located frontally and parietally. In cases of seizures in elderly patients (>70 years), suspicious lesions in the brain usually are metastasis, glioma, or CNS lymphoma (in order of decreasing frequency).[32]

MRI easily demonstrates the origin of seizures but may show other causes of seizure in a cancer patient, such as meningitis or brain abscess, radiation necrosis, thrombocytopenia associated intracranial hemorrhage, or lesions suggesting a limbic (paraneoplastic) encephalitis. The latter is commonly associated with seizures and nonconvulsive or convulsive status epilepticus. Chemotherapy can cause seizures, mostly through severe electrolyte abnormalities (Table 9.1). When many drugs are administered, large fluid volumes may precipitate a severe hyponatremia, and patients with cancer-related lingering SIADH are most susceptible to abrupt changes.

Table 9.1 **Chemotherapy Drugs that Cause Seizures Through Acute Electrolytic Abnormalities**

Drug	Abnormality
Cisplatin	Hypomagnesemia
Cyclophosphamide, oxcarbazepine	Hyponatremia
Cisplatin	Hypocalcemia

Focal new deficits are also common; they usually represent a new hemiparesis, visual field deficit, language difficulty, or ataxia when associated with lesions in the cerebellum. Some of these symptoms are related to brain edema surrounding the lesion and will markedly improve with high-dose corticosteroids. New presence of hemorrhage into a metastasis may also produce acute focal findings (e.g., hemiparesis, speech impairment). In some cases, these hemorrhages can fully overshadow the malignant lesion, which is usually diagnosed after neurosurgical extirpation.

Decrease in responsiveness may be related to three causes: (1) metastasis in the thalamus interrupting thalamocortical traffic, (2) mass effect with brainstem displacement causing thalamic compression or dysfunction of the ascending reticular formation, and (3) development of obstructive hydrocephalus causing stupor. In many of these patients, there is a prior history of poor cognitive functioning before alertness became compromised.

A solitary mass in the cerebellum may cause marked displacement of the brainstem. Removal is considered good palliation because the patient becomes more communicative and able to voice his or her wishes. In other situations, care depends entirely on the presence of other intracranial or extracranial metastatic lesions—and some neurosurgeons opt not to intervene with surgery or even a ventriculostomy. Metastasis in the spinal cord can cause acute hydrocephalus due to blockade of CSF circulation in the spinal area, and MRI may be needed if no cranial lesions are seen.

A consult may be requested for pain management or evaluation if a neuropathic pain is present. Neurologic pain is less common, and the pain mechanism often primarily relates to bone involvement. Pain associated with acute neuropathies (plexopathies, radiculopathies, or polyneuropathies) is predominantly associated with dysesthesias (positive symptoms of painful tingling) and hypesthesias (areas of sensory loss), but severe stabbing and burning pain can occur with any nerve involvement. Carcinomatous meningitis may be associated with relentless extremity and back pain. Acute pain in a cancer patient is not a reason for admission to the ICU, but often its treatment with opioids is the main culprit. Occasionally, patients are admitted with respiratory arrest, particularly opioid-naïve patients.

LEPTOMENINGEAL METASTASIS

Leptomeningeal metastasis is a major terminal complication of cancer. Although the clinical features can be protracted, with headache and confusion at presentation, many patients develop cranial nerve deficits. Multiple cranial nerve involvement in a patient with known cancer is likely leptomeningeal seeding. This complication is seen with increasing frequency in ICU patients, most commonly in those with carcinomas or hematologic cancers such as non-Hodgkin's lymphomas and leukemias. Melanoma, breast cancer, and SCLC are common solid tumors that cause metastasis to the meninges. Primary lymphoid meningitis has also been reported, but onset is more insidious—it is also very responsive to methotrexate treatment.[34]

Next to cranial nerve deficits, loss of vision is more common than is appreciated in neoplastic meningitis. Involvement of oropharyngeal function resulting in loss of the gag reflex and swallowing is a common reason for endotracheal intubation.

Leukemias and lymphomas that involve the meninges are typically treated with intrathecal or systemic chemotherapy, and often with adjunctive radiotherapy. Some of these patients need to have chemotherapy administered into the CSF by means of an Ommaya device. The chemotherapy agents most commonly used in the treatment of leptomeningeal metastases are shown in Table 9.2.[13] Many patients relapse months after the diagnosis despite treatment.

BRAIN METASTASES

Acute hemorrhage into a brain metastasis or the development of lymphoma resulting in brain metastases and cerebral edema may bring a patient to the ICU. Treatment

Table 9.2 **Chemotherapy Agents Used to Treat Leptomeningeal Metastasis**

Drug	Mode of delivery	Primary cancer
Methotrexate	Systemic IV Intra-CSF	Lymphoma, solid tumors
Cytarabine	Intra-CSF	Lymphoma, solid tumors
Lapatinib	Systemic oral	Breast (HER2-positive)
Gefitinib	Systemic oral	NSCLC (EGFR-mutated)
Capecitabine	Systemic oral	Breast, lung
Bevacizumab	Systemic IV	Colorectal, lung, renal, glioblastoma
Rituximab	Systemic IV Intra-CSF	Lymphoma

CSF, cerebrospinal fluid; HER2, human epidermal growth factor receptor 2; EGFR, epidermal growth factor receptor; NSCLC, non–small-cell lung cancer. Not all indications have been approved by the US Food and Drug Administration.

Adapted from Grewal et al.[14]

is with high-dose corticosteroids, but in many patients progression occurs despite management.[9,11,12,25] The tumor that originally is responsible for the brain metastases may determine the clinical course and prognosis. (Melanomas have a higher incidence of hemorrhage into metastases, as do HER2-positive breast cancers.[35]) Further targeted therapy includes resection and radiation.[31] The most aggressive approach would be to combine stereotactic radiosurgery with whole-brain irradiation, particularly if surgery is not possible in eloquent locations. There is a concern about increased toxicity with the combination, and a targeted approach may have a similar effect. Median survival time is an estimated 10–12 months for small multiple metastases but more rapid demise if mass effect is seen.

PRIMARY CENTRAL NERVOUS SYSTEM LYMPHOMA

There is an increasing prevalence of CNS lymphoma in elderly patients, though this is still a rare brain tumor in comparison to all other CNS tumors (<3%).[23] Lymphoma can involve the brain or spinal cord preferentially. Almost all of these tumors are large B-cell lymphomas. Most patients have a history of gradual personality change, but an acute presentation (progressive headache or seizures) may occur. On computed tomography, the lesions are hypodense and scattered throughout; they are hypo intense on T1-weighted MRI and with gadolinium administration diffuse, homogeneous contrast-enhancement is expected.[6] DWI may be restricted in these highly cellular tumors, differentiating it from astrocytomas.

Therapeutic options are systemic methotrexate with whole-brain radiotherapy, which may lead to some relief of symptoms.[28] I have seen three fulminant cases with coma at presentation that progressed despite high doses of corticosteroids (Figure 9-3). Others have observed dramatic improvement with corticosteroids, but only if there are no clinical signs of brainstem displacement or increased intracranial pressure causing impaired consciousness.[10] Outcome can be poor (<50% survival at 2 years) if there are multiple factors, low performance status at diagnosis, elevated

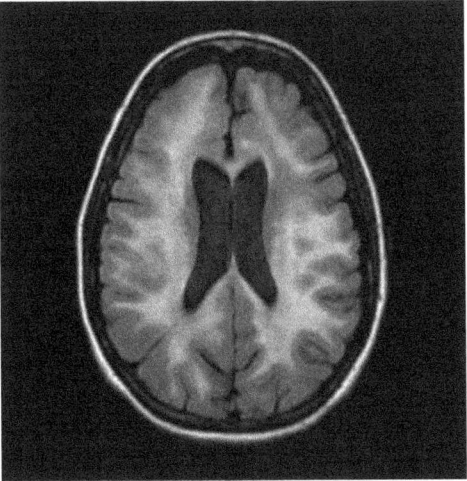

Figure 9.3 MRI shows primary CNS lymphoma.

serum lactate dehydrogenase, high CSF protein concentration, and tumor location within the deep regions of the brain (e.g., periventricular region, basal ganglia, brainstem).

PARANEOPLASTIC SYNDROMES

Another commonly seen complication is an acute paraneoplastic manifestation of cancer. (Further details can be found in another volume in this series, *Handling Difficult Situations*.) Many patients with paraneoplastic hemispheric syndrome have focal seizures or nonconvulsive status epilepticus at presentation. In some patients, the basal ganglia and thalami are involved, and this can produce a marked change in level of consciousness. Major syndromes that have been described are limbic encephalitis, bulbar (brainstem) encephalitis, and cerebellar encephalitis and all may be associated with a myelitis. Patients who have a brainstem encephalitis have major eye findings (e.g., opsoclonus) at presentation. This symptomatology can rapidly progress, and patients may become increasingly stuporous, but they may also develop marked hypoventilation and a need for intubation. Extensive involvement of the brainstem is usually seen on MRI. In most instances of limbic encephalitis, patients present with unusual new agitated behavior, often punctuated by a seizure. Most patients with paraneoplastic limbic encephalitis do not only have an affective disorder but also neurobehavioral abnormalities such as apraxia, aphasia, acalculia, and visual recognition abnormalities. Some have more specific characteristics. The anti-Ma2 encephalitis is associated with daytime sleepiness and narcolepsy in about one third of patients. (Testicular tumors are common in anti-Ma2 encephalitis.)

Paraneoplastic syndromes are often associated with positive antibodies such as anti-Yo or anti-Hu, which are linked with ovarian cancer and SCLC, respectively. Aggressive immunosuppression with corticosteroids or intravenous immunoglobulin may result in a response, although in some patients, plasma exchange or a combination of rituximab and cyclophosphamide may be needed. In general, the response to immunotherapy is poor (Table 9.3).[30]

STROKE RELATED TO CANCER

Stroke may be caused by coagulation abnormalities and is predominantly seen in patients with hematologic malignancies who are admitted to the ICU. As expected, the appearance of acute thrombocytopenia may lead to acute hemorrhages in the CNS, and hematology-oncology disorders predominate in cases of coagulopathy-associated cerebral hemorrhage. Cerebral hemorrhage in the acute leukemias is mostly a consequence of thrombocytopenia, alone or from leukemic infiltrates. Intracerebral hematoma is caused by hemorrhage in a metastasis and can result from invasion of vessel walls or dura by tumor causing neoplastic subdural hemorrhage (commonly seen with gastric, prostate, and breast cancers, but also with leukemias). Hemorrhages

Table 9.3 **Classic Paraneoplastic Neurologic Syndromes**

Syndrome	Cancer associations	Antineuronal antibody	Response to immunotherapy
Encephalomyelitis	SCLC	Anti-Hu	Poor
Encephalomyelitis, uveitis, peripheral neuropathy	SCLC, thymoma	Anti-CV2/CRMP5	Poor
Subacute sensory neuronopathy	SCLC, others	Anti-Hu with SCLC but not other solid tumors	Poor
Limbic, brainstem, hypothalamic encephalitis	Testicular germ-cell tumors	Anti-Ma2	Response in 30%
Cerebellar degeneration	Gynecologic, breast	Anti-Yo	Poor
Cerebellar degeneration, opsoclonus	Gynecologic, breast	Anti-Ri	Poor
Cerebellar degeneration	Hodgkin's lymphoma	Anti-Tr	Response in 20%
Stiff-man syndrome, encephalomyelitis	Breast, SCLC	Anti-amphiphysin	Reports of some response
Opsoclonus-myoclonus	Neuroblastoma in children; various solid tumors in adults	Anti-Ri is found in a subset of women with breast or gynecologic cancers	Variable

CRMP5, collapsin response mediator protein 5; SCLC, small-cell lung cancer.

Adapted from Rosenfeld and Dalmau.[30]

can be single or in multiple compartments, small and petechial, or quite sizable and destructive.

Treatment consists of immediate platelet transfusion and often neurosurgical evacuation if mass effect is present. Neurosurgical intervention is rarely successful, because platelet infusion to correct a major thrombocytopenia takes time and many patients deteriorate significantly before intervention. Many chemotherapeutic agents (often used in combination) can lead to thrombocytopenia. Bevacizumab (used to treat non-SCLC and colon cancer) may cause hemorrhagic infarctions, and the risk is higher if it is used in combination with other chemotherapeutic agents.

At the other end of the spectrum of neoplastic coagulopathies is systemic thrombosis, which may result in microthrombi in cerebral arterioles. Prothrombotic states are common in solid tumors and in hematologic malignancies, but hyperviscosity syndromes may appear with massive increases in leukocyte counts (>100,000/mm^3). Moreover, in patients with advanced metastatic cancer, disseminated intravascular coagulation or nonbacterial thrombotic endocarditis may occur (the latter more common in pancreatic cancer). These are all urgent conditions—many overlapping—and can lead to cerebral infarction. Therapeutic options for ischemic stroke are limited to intravenous heparin and later rehabilitation, but only if the patient's general condition allows such intervention. Other systemic emboli are often seen, and this is a major terminal complication. With increased use of endovascular procedures for selective administration of antineoplastic drugs, complications may increase, but the incidence of ischemic stroke is low.

CENTRAL NERVOUS SYSTEMS INFECTIONS IN CANCER

This complication may lead to medical ICU admission, but more often in immunocompromised patients and in those who have undergone hematopoietic stem cell transplantation (see another volume in this series, *Handling Difficult Situations*). A few practical concluding remarks here.

Organisms to consider are *Aspergillus*, cryptococcus and candida, listeria, tuberculosis, and three viruses (JC virus, varicella zoster virus [VZV], and Epstein–Barr virus). Neurosurgical procedures (biopsy and debulking) increase the risk for *Staphylococcus aureus* infection, meningitis, and ventriculitis. In hematopoietic stem cell transplantation, infectious complications may be related to the time from transplantation: from 0 to 1 months; they are more likely to be caused by cytomegalovirus (CMV), *Aspergillus*, or human herpesvirus 6—from 1–12 months; infections may be due to by herpes simplex virus, VZV, and CMV reactivation.

Putting It All Together

- ICU consultation for neurologic complications of cancer usually involves a new metastasis or worsening from leptomeningeal seeding.
- Management of a neurooncologic complication may be effective, albeit palliative.
- Acute metabolic derangements and tumor lysis syndrome can cause neurologic manifestations.
- Chemotherapy may cause some neurologic complications.
- Coagulopathies often cause strokes (hemorrhagic and ischemic).

> **By the Way**
>
> - Neoplastic meningitis may be mimicked by infections.
> - Procedures may increase the risk of CNS complications.
> - Brain metastasis may lead to obstruction of CSF, requiring ventriculostomy.
> - Autoimmune encephalitis is associated with ovarian cancer in females.

> **Neurooncologic Emergencies by the Numbers**
>
> - ~50% of brain metastases originate from lung cancer.
> - ~50% of patients with limbic encephalitis have demonstrable neuronal antibodies.
> - ~20% of hematologic malignancies have CSF seeding.
> - ~15% of solid tumors result in leptomeningeal metastases.
> - ~5% of patients with chemotherapy develop acute leukoencephalopathy.

References

1. Aygencel G, Turkoglu M, Turkoz Sucak G, Benekli M. Prognostic factors in critically ill cancer patients admitted to the intensive care unit. *J Crit Care* 2014;29:618–626.
2. Beauchesne P. Intrathecal chemotherapy for treatment of leptomeningeal dissemination of metastatic tumours. *Lancet Oncol* 2010;11:871–879.
3. Bernal T, Pardavila EV, Bonastre J, et al. Survival of hematological patients after discharge from the intensive care unit: a prospective observational study. *Crit Care* 2013;17:R302.
4. Bird GT, Farquhar-Smith P, Wigmore T, Potter M, Gruber PC. Outcomes and prognostic factors in patients with hematological malignancy admitted to a specialist cancer intensive care unit: a 5 yr study. *Br J Anaesth* 2012;108:452–459.
5. Bos MM, de Keizer NF, Meynaar IA, Bakhshi-Raiez F, de Jonge E. Outcomes of cancer patients after unplanned admission to general intensive care units. *Acta Oncol* 2012;51:897–905.
6. Coulon A, Lafitte F, Hoang-Xuan K, et al. Radiographic findings in 37 cases of primary CNS lymphoma in immunocompetent patients. *Eur Radiol* 2002;12:329–340.
7. Darnell RB, Posner JB. *Paraneoplastic Syndromes*. New York: Oxford University Press, 2011.
8. DeAngelis LM, Posner JB. *Neurologic Complications of Cancer*: Oxford: Oxford University Press, 2009.
9. Delattre JY, Krol G, Thaler HT, Posner JB. Distribution of brain metastases. *Arch Neurol* 1988;45:741–744.
10. Finsterer J, Lubec D, Jellinger K, Mamoli B. Recovery from coma caused by primary CNS mantle cell lymphoma presenting as encephalitis. *Neurology* 1996;46:824–826.
11. Gallego Perez-Larraya J, Hildebrand J. Brain metastases. *Handb Clin Neurol* 2014;121:1143–1157.
12. Gavrilovic IT, Posner JB. Brain metastases: epidemiology and pathophysiology. *J Neurooncol* 2005;75:5–14.
13. Gleissner B, Chamberlain MC. Neoplastic meningitis. *Lancet Neurol* 2006;5:443–452.
14. Grewal J, Saria MG, Kesari S. Novel approaches to treating leptomeningeal metastases. *J Neurooncol* 2012;106:225–234.

15. Hoff AO, Vassilopoulou-Sellin R. The role of glucagon administration in the diagnosis and treatment of patients with tumor hypoglycemia. *Cancer* 1998;82:1585–1592.
16. Kaito E, Terae S, Kobayashi R, et al. The role of tumor lysis in reversible posterior leukoencephalopathy syndrome. *Pediatr Radiol* 2005;35:722–727.
17. Kouroukis TC, Baldassarre FG, Haynes AE, et al. Bortezomib in multiple myeloma: systematic review and clinical considerations. *Curr Oncol* 2014;21:e573–e603.
18. Lin YC, Tsai YH, Huang CC, et al. Outcome of lung cancer patients with acute respiratory failure requiring mechanical ventilation. *Respir Med* 2004;98:43–51.
19. McGrath S, Chatterjee F, Whiteley C, Ostermann M. ICU and 6-month outcome of oncology patients in the intensive care unit. *QJM* 2010;103:397–403.
20. Naeem N, Reed MD, Creger RJ, Youngner SJ, Lazarus HM. Transfer of the hematopoietic stem cell transplant patient to the intensive care unit: does it really matter? *Bone Marrow Transplant* 2006;37:119–133.
21. Nazer LH, Hawari F, Al-Najjar T. Adverse drug events in critically ill patients with cancer: incidence, characteristics, and outcomes. *J Pharm Pract* 2014;27:208–213.
22. O'Meara WP, Borkar SA, Stambuk HE, Lymberis SC. Leptomeningeal metastasis. *Curr Probl Cancer* 2007;31:367–424.
23. O'Neill BP, Decker PA, Tieu C, Cerhan JR. The changing incidence of primary central nervous system lymphoma is driven primarily by the changing incidence in young and middle-aged men and differs from time trends in systemic diffuse large B-cell non-Hodgkin's lymphoma. *Am J Hematol* 2013;88:997–1000.
24. Ozcan C, Wong SJ, Hari P. Reversible posterior leukoencephalopathy syndrome and bevacizumab. *N Engl J Med* 2006;354:980–982.
25. Patchell RA. The management of brain metastases. *Cancer Treat Rev* 2003;29:533–540.
26. Pauls S, Fischer AC, Brambs HJ, et al. Use of magnetic resonance imaging to detect neoplastic meningitis: limited use in leukemia and lymphoma but convincing results in solid tumors. *Eur J Radiol* 2012;81:974–978.
27. Pelosof LC, Gerber DE. Paraneoplastic syndromes: an approach to diagnosis and treatment. *Mayo Clin Proc* 2010;85:838–854.
28. Phillips EH, Fox CP, Cwynarski K. Primary CNS lymphoma. *Curr Hematol Malig Rep* 2014;9:243–253.
29. Raftopoulos H. Diagnosis and management of hyponatremia in cancer patients. *Support Care Cancer* 2007;15:1341–1347.
30. Rosenfeld MR, Dalmau J. Diagnosis and management of paraneoplastic neurologic disorders. *Curr Treat Options Oncol* 2013;14:528–538.
31. Ruskin R, Urban RR, Sherman AE, et al. Predictors of intensive care unit utilization in gynecologic oncology surgery. *Int J Gynecol Cancer* 2011;21:1336–1342.
32. Schiff D, Kesari S, Wen PCY. *Cancer Neurology in Clinical Practice: Neurologic Complications of Cancer and Its Treatment.* 2nd ed. New York: Humana Press, 2008.
33. Schwartz WB, Bennett W, Curelop S, Bartter FC. A syndrome of renal sodium loss and hyponatremia probably resulting from inappropriate secretion of antidiuretic hormone. *Am J Med* 1957;23:529–542.
34. Shapiro WR, Johanson CE, Boogerd W. Treatment modalities for leptomeningeal metastases. *Semin Oncol* 2009;36:S46–S54.
35. Shen Q, Sahin AA, Hess KR, et al. Breast cancer with brain metastases: clinicopathologic features, survival, and paired biomarker analysis. *Oncologist* 2015;20:466-473.
36. Slatore CG, Cecere LM, Letourneau JL, et al. Intensive care unit outcomes among patients with lung cancer in the surveillance, epidemiology, and end results Medicare registry. *J Clin Oncol* 2012;30:1686–1691.
37. Soffietti R, Trevisan E, Ruda R. Neurologic complications of chemotherapy and other newer and experimental approaches. *Handb Clin Neurol* 2014;121:1199–1218.
38. Song JU, Suh GY, Park HY, et al. Early intervention on the outcomes in critically ill cancer patients admitted to intensive care units. *Intensive Care Med* 2012;38:1505–1513.

39. Tam CS, Galanos J, Seymour JF, et al. Reversible posterior leukoencephalopathy syndrome complicating cytotoxic chemotherapy for hematologic malignancies. *Am J Hematol* 2004;77:72–76.
40. Vaughn C, Zhang L, Schiff D. Reversible posterior leukoencephalopathy syndrome in cancer. *Curr Oncol Rep* 2008;10:86–91.
41. Verstappen CC, Heimans JJ, Hoekman K, Postma TJ. Neurotoxic complications of chemotherapy in patients with cancer: clinical signs and optimal management. *Drugs* 2003;63:1549–1563.
42. Windebank AJ, Grisold W. Chemotherapy-induced neuropathy. *J Peripher Nerv Syst* 2008;13:27–46.
43. Zedan AH, Vilholm OJ. Chemotherapy-induced polyneuropathy: major agents and assessment by questionnaires. *Basic Clin Pharmacol Toxicol* 2014;115:193–200.

10

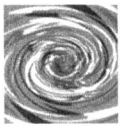

Troubleshooting: ICU Neurotoxicology

Each year, medical intensive care units (ICUs) have a considerable number of patients who have intentionally overdosed. Many of them are deeply comatose and have been intubated when it was found they could not protect the airway, but others are markedly agitated and jittery and in a full-blown delirium. It is not uncommon to see a patient with a self-inflicted intoxication and a flurry of seizures who requires the immediate use of high-dose benzodiazepines and other anticonvulsants. Abrupt onset of seizures in young children who have been exploring their parents' medications must first point to salicylates. In adults, antidepressants remain the easiest drug to get when suicidal. Suicidal ingestion in adults is a common cause of intoxications, and physicians are often misled by the seriousness of the attempt. There are some unusual ingestions. For example, isoniazid, which is a notorious cause of toxicity in places with a high prevalence of tuberculosis.

Intoxications and medication overdoses can be immediately problematic and may lead to a permanent neurologic deficit. In many instances, the clinical presentation cannot easily be attributed to a single known toxin. Some adolescents have been very successful in their attempt (not always willingly and intentionally), and anoxic-ischemic injury to the brain may have already occurred before transfer.

This chapter does not focus, however, on the specific management of poisonings—there are very few, and some of the diagnostic challenges and use of antidotes are described in another volume in this series, *Handling Difficult Situations*. Instead, it concentrates on how the neurologist can be useful in assessment of the severity of the intoxication and in its management, particularly when there are recurrent seizures or permanent loss of consciousness. The neurologist is typically consulted when, for some reason, the intensivist feels that the toxin has lingered too long and coma cannot be explained by decreased elimination or prolonged absorption. Furthermore, by the time the neurologist sees the patient, most principles of detoxification should be in effect, including gastric decontamination resulting in enhanced elimination of the drug, hemodialysis in some patients for active removal (e.g., salicylate, lithium), urine alkalinization to improve elimination, and specific antidotes to reduce the effect of the poison or toxin.

There is an outside world of drug abusers, intentional poisoners, and even victims of chemical terrorism. Several major cities in the United States have a major heroin problem. Self-poisoning with prescribed medication is most prevalent, but Poison Control Centers help to facilitate recognition of unusual poisons in unexplained presentations. Therefore, the most important questions that the consulting neurologist should ask are the following: Is there a specific toxidrome that could point in a certain direction? Are there elements of permanent injury, particularly anoxic-ischemic injury? Would a magnetic resonance imaging (MRI) scan be helpful? Does the patient need continuous electroencephalography (EEG) monitoring for recognition and management of ongoing seizures?

Experience with treatment of toxic exposures cannot be expected, even for the practiced intensivist. With some variation, ICU population studies include fewer than 5% of patients with intoxications, and large numbers of similar intoxications may rarely occur. Accredited medical toxicologists (accessible by telephone at 1-800-222-1222 in the United States) are therefore necessary to provide the much-needed expertise.[6–8,11]

Fortunately, many patients will improve and awaken within 24 hours after admission and no sequelae are found. Many are subsequently transferred to a psychiatric unit for further care. This is not always the case. Mortality is substantially (sixfold) higher in patients using street drugs when there is long-term follow-up after hospital discharge.[1,2] Many of these individuals believe that some day they will straighten up, but they don't and are readmitted at some point. For some addicts, loss of tolerance during hospital admission and resumption of drug use at prior dose levels result in a deadly outcome.

Intoxications with antidepressants (particularly selective serotonin reuptake inhibitors [SSRIs]) have increased, and intoxications with benzodiazepines have decreased. In the largest study to date (>7,000 ICU patients), combinations of alcohol and sedatives were found 22% of the time, and antidepressants and sedatives 17% of the time.[1] In this chapter we will review intoxications causing neurologic manifestations.

The Overdosed Patient

The typical overdosed patient in the ICU has taken sedatives or a combination of drugs.[1] Mortality is generally low, because many of these drugs do not cause multiorgan failure or result in persistent coma. Even if aspiration occurs or there is a sudden increase in creatine phosphokinase or liver enzymes, the patient is often young (30–40 years), intrinsically healthy, and able to overcome this insult to major organ systems. Intubation, mechanical ventilation, and waiting out clearance of the toxin may be all there is to it. Not infrequently, a nonurgent neurology consult is placed, but by the next day, the drug has cleared and the patient is groggy, bewildered, and sometimes apologetic. However, it can be far more serious and typical clinical manifestations of some of the most common intoxications are shown in Figure 10.1. A simple classification may help orient the physician when it comes to type of intoxication (Table 10.1).

Toxidromes—the toxicology syndromes—consist of combinations of key vital signs: blood pressure, pulse rate, respiratory rate, temperature, pupil size, peristalsis, and texture of the skin. Rarely does an intoxication or poisoning perfectly

Troubleshooting: ICU Neurotoxicology 139

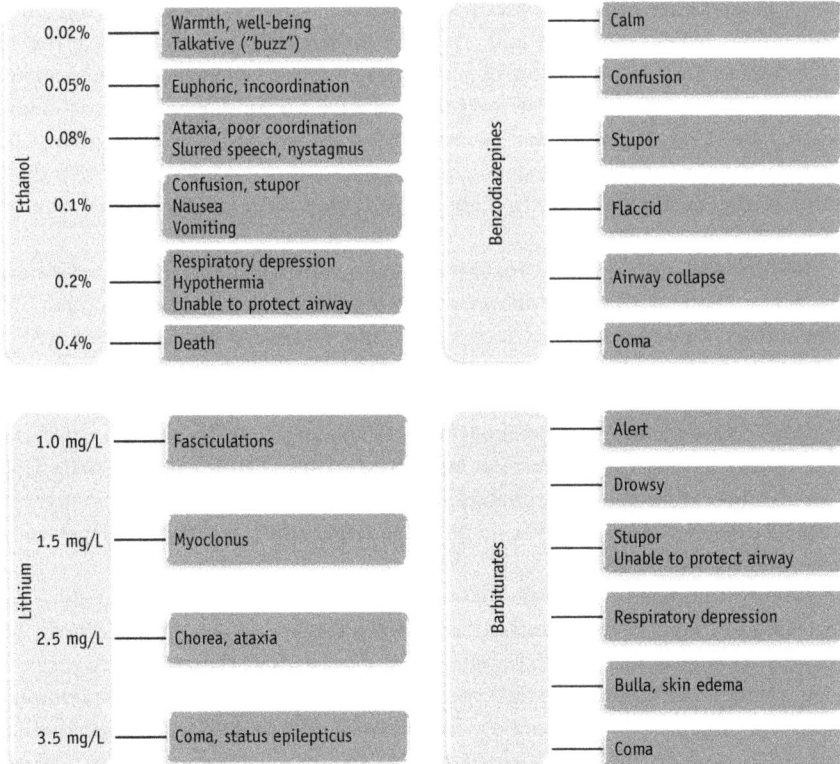

Figure 10.1 Symptoms and signs of four major common intoxications. (Data from Nelson et al.[15])

include all elements of these toxidromes. It is a common error to attribute the severity of the intoxication to the number of manifestations. Often manifestations are a consequence of a single physiologic change (e.g., volume depletion induced by sweating that leads to hypotension or pulse rate that changes as a result of temperature change). Respiration is the most difficult factor to assess, because

Table 10.1 **Categorization of Intoxications**

- Alcohol
- Analgesics (salicylates, acetaminophen)
- Antidepressants (tricyclic antidepressants, SSRIs, lithium)
- Street drugs (heroin, cocaine, amphetamines)
- Sedatives (benzodiazepines, antipsychotics)
- Poisons (carbon monoxide, arsenic, cyanide)
- Miscellaneous
- Combinations

SSRIs, selective serotonin reuptake inhibitors.

many patients are intubated and their respiratory rate is ventilator-controlled. Continuous hyperventilation and a patient consistently breathing above the set rate can result from ingestion of atypical alcohols or salicylates. Temperature assessment (though only in the extremes) is very helpful for pinpointing culprit toxins. However, hypothermia is common in any elderly, frail, and poorly fed patient (due to decreased temperature discrimination and decreased metabolic rate), as well as in patients with diabetes, or it may occur simply because of environmental factors.

Another stipulation is that toxidromes are not perfectly specific for toxins and likewise remain uncommonly observed. Sympathomimetic toxidrome pictures (i.e., diaphoresis, dilated pupil, and tachycardia) can be seen in thyrotoxicosis and in alcohol withdrawal syndrome. A cholinergic toxidrome (i.e., myosis, fasciculation, salivation, hypertension, tachycardia, and sweating) is seen with organophosphates and thus a rare occurrence. The opposite, anticholinergic toxidrome (i.e., mydriasis, tremors, hypertension, tachycardia, and dry skin) may be seen with toxicity from scopolamine, atropine, or antihistamines, but this also is an unusual occurrence. Cyclic antidepressants can cause an anticholinergic effect, but the antidepressants now used are mostly SSRIs.

Sympathicomimetic toxidrome is seen with use of cocaine (all vital signs are increased, resulting in hypertension, tachycardia, tachypnea, and hyperthermia). The symptomatology of cocaine use is well known, along with its characteristics.

It is important to recognize the hyperthermic syndromes, which include serotonin syndrome, neuroleptic malignant syndrome, and especially malignant hyperthermia (Table 10.2).[15,16] An uncommon syndrome that should be known and (hopefully) recognized is neuroleptic malignant syndrome, which is caused by dopamine antagonists. Patients often have hyperthermia and marked rigidity, but also dysautonomia and hypotension alternating with hypertension.

The serotonin syndrome, caused by overdose of SSRIs, usually manifests with agitation, akathisia, tachycardia, and myoclonus. All patients are stuporous, and some become comatose. Additional use of opioids, particularly fentanyl and antiemetics, may precipitate serotonin syndrome or worsen its manifestations.[15]

A general rule is that impaired consciousness and coma are more often seen with abuse of sympathicolytics, opioids, and sedatives. Restlessness, agitation,

Table 10.2 **Drugs or Toxins that Affect Core Temperature**

Hyperthermia (>38°C)	*Hypothermia (<35°C)*
Anticholinergics	Ethanol
Neuroleptics	Hypoglycemics
SSRIs	Sedatives
Sympathicomimetics	α-Adrenergic agonists
Salicylates	Carbon monoxide

SSRIs, selective serotonin reuptake inhibitors.

and delirium are more often seen with sympathicomimetics, anticholinergics, and hallucinogens.

Because of their high mortality rate (30%–40%), the most important toxins that need to be recognized are the atypical alcohols, such as ethylene glycol and methanol. They cause an increased anion gap (>2 mEq/L), and they also increase the osmolar gap (>10 mOsm/L). Finding this combination (wide anion gap metabolic acidosis plus elevated osmolar gap) often points to ingestion of an atypical alcohol, and its presence is a strong indication for blockade of its effects by fomepizole. It is a reminder that every suspected intoxication needs to be evaluated with an arterial blood gas analysis.

Toxicology screening is useful, but every physician is trained to appreciate its major limitations, and many drugs are not screened for presence or serum levels (Table 10.3). Each hospital laboratory may develop its own focused toxicology screens, typically including barbiturates, acetaminophen, alcohols, salicylates, and tricyclic antidepressants.

Treatment of any intoxication rests on supporting or correcting the major vital signs—some patients are critically and near fatally poisoned. Damage can be devastating and permanent, not only to the brain but also to kidneys and liver. The neurologic manifestations may be markedly confounded by acute renal shutdown or fulminant hepatic necrosis. Fluid resuscitation and cooling devices are required to reduce hyperthermia. Bradycardia is treated when hypotension occurs. Severe hypotension may require vasopressors. Transvenous pacemaker placement, intraaortic balloon pump, and even extracorporeal membrane oxygenation may be needed if bradycardia is refractory. General measures of perfusion, such as urinary output and serum lactate levels, remain good initial guides.

Supportive care is needed in most of the less critical intoxications that are commonly seen. Other adjunctive measures are needed. For example, in alcohol intoxication, one can expect poor nutritional status, and patients are treated immediately with intravenous thiamine (100 mg daily) as well as dextrose solutions to prevent a

Table 10.3 **Important Intoxications Not Detected by Most Toxicology Screens**

Antiepileptics
Antipsychotics
Serotonin reuptake inhibitors
Methanol and ethylene glycol
Lithium
Calcium channel blockers and β-blockers
Fentanyl
Clonidine
Solvents
Strychnine

From Nelson LS, Levin NA, Howland MA, et al., eds. *Goldfrank's Toxicologic Emergencies*. 9th edition. New York: McGraw-Hill, 2011.

hypoglycemia that could cause a severe brain injury if not recognized. Alcohol intoxication followed by Wernicke–Korsakoff syndrome is not common, but can occur if the patient is given intravenous glucose and insufficient thiamine. Failure to awaken, or slow awakening with marked ophthalmoparesis, is a key neurologic feature.

Principles of Neurotoxicology

How does a toxin damage the brain? The main mechanisms for reversible neurotoxicity involve temporary interruption or stimulation of neurotransmitter effects. Seizures are a result of such excitation (excitotoxicity). Impairment of consciousness occurs through enhancement of γ-aminobutyric acid neurotransmission. Marked movement disorders occur through damage of dopaminergic neurons in the basal ganglia, but glutamatergic and cholinergic neurons participate in the process as well. This knowledge may not be clinically relevant because secondary damage resulting from marked hypotension and hypoxemia could determine the injury. Acute additional liver and kidney injuries may confound the neurologic examination. Who does not remember the markedly intoxicated teenager found comatose (hypotensive and hypoventilating) the next day by his friends who checked up on him after they let him sleep for the entire morning?

A major example is heroin overdose, which in 1 of 10 patients causes pulmonary edema due to acute respiratory distress syndrome that may manifest emergently and cause severe hypoxemia—all resulting in infarcts in the globus pallidus. Inhaled heroin can cause status asthmaticus. Injected heroin can cause embolization of particulate matter, but more likely the mechanism is toxic vasculitis or in extreme circumstances a hypertensive emergency leading to cerebral hemorrhage, often in typical ganglionic locations.

Amphetamine abuse is also notorious for cerebral hemorrhage, and ischemic stroke may occur as a result of necrotizing vasculitis in long-term users. Cerebral angiograms in patients with amphetamine use have shown beading and end-artery cutoffs.

Accidental ingestion of a high dose of calcium channel blockers may result in a near-fatal clinical toxicity. The cardiac affects are prominent, causing hypotension largely due to vasodilatation. In most patients, an increasing heart block is followed by junctional bradycardia and, eventually, asystole. Toxicity due to calcium channel blockers can cause rapid deterioration; patients may quickly become critically ill and their condition difficult to manage. Calcium channel blockers affect dopaminergic systems, which may lead to multifocal myoclonus in facial muscles and extremities. This cannot be differentiated from myoclonus associated with severe anoxic-ischemic injury except that many patients are responsive to questions and not comatose.

TRANSIENT NEUROTOXICOLOGIC SYMPTOMS

The toxins that should not cause permanent neurologic injury (unless the patient arrives in shock after being found apneic) are benzodiazepines, barbiturates, antidepressants, lithium, antipsychotic drugs, and calcium channel blockers.

Again, alcohol intoxication rarely causes major problems except in a naïve drinker. Ethanol-induced ketoacidosis can also be fatal. Cases of ethanol intoxication are notorious for co-ingestion of illicit drugs and association with brawls leading to traumatic brain and spine injuries. Most of the time is spent excluding significant cervical spine injury, fractures, or traumatic brain injury; this may require computed tomography, MRI, and a large number of other radiologic studies. Usually, blood alcohol levels are measured on a "per mil" (‰) basis, which is equivalent to mg/dL divided by 1,000. In general, blood alcohol levels of 4‰ (i.e., 0.4%) or higher can lead to respiratory arrest, but chronic alcoholics may survive three times higher percentages.

A common error is attributing a decreased level of consciousness to alcohol intoxication in a previously known alcoholic and therefore neglecting to perform an examination of the cerebrospinal fluid for bacterial meningitis. This should be considered if the blood alcohol level is relatively low for what is seen clinically, again assuming tolerance for alcohol. The symptoms and effects of alcohol intoxication in more or less naïve or incidental drinkers are shown in Figure 10.1. Some patients have an alcohol-induced hypoglycemia that manifests with hyperthermia and tachypnea, but rehydration is usually successful, and prolonged sequelae are rarely found. The situation becomes problematic if the patient fails to awaken or if there are other persistent neurologic signs.

Some patients have rapidly evolving neurologic symptomatology that seems to worsen by the hour. A typical example is lithium overdose in the setting of a suicide attempt. Usually, toxicity is defined as a blood lithium level of 1.5 mEq/L or higher. Patients initially become agitated and then develop fasciculations and ataxia, rapidly followed by seizures. Severe myoclonus status epilepticus may be seen in lithium intoxication and cannot be differentiated clinically from myoclonus status epilepticus in postresuscitation encephalopathy. The management may include peritoneal dialysis or hemodialysis, particularly in patients who have recurrent seizures. Seizures are treated with a combination of benzodiazepines and phenytoin without any later concerns. Fasciculations and choreiform movements are also typical. Hemodialysis is needed if epileptiform activity is seen on EEG.[13,18,20] Lithium overdose can result in permanent kidney injury, but many patients do well. Usually, blood lithium levels must be greater than 2.5 mEq/L to result in coma.

Benzodiazepines predominate as causes for intoxications in the medical ICU. Flumazenil (0.2 mg IV and repeated doses) is usually considered, but its effect is short-lived, because many patients have ingested long-acting benzodiazepines (e.g., clonazepam, diazepam). Even when other drugs are co-ingested, the effect is transient. It may take 1 or 2 days before patients are able to adequately protect their airway.

Barbiturates may result in far more systemic effects due to myocardial depression. Full ICU support to allow washout is the best option. Measurement of barbiturate levels can guide clinicians as to when extubation might be expected (usually, pentobarbital <1 mg/mL and phenobarbital <15 mg/mL).

The agitated intoxicated patient often has an anticholinergic or sympathomimetic toxidrome (or a *forme fruste*). These toxidromes are similar in causing tachycardia and hyperthermia, but patients with a sympathomimetic toxidrome are said to be "wet," with very moist axillae, whereas those with an anticholinergic toxidrome are dry ("dry

Table 10.4 **Drugs that Exacerbate Serotonin Syndrome associated with Selective Serotonin Reuptake Inhibitors**

Lithium
Antiepileptics (valproate)
Antiemetics (ondansetron, metoclopramide)
Antimigraine drugs (sumatriptan)
Antibiotics (linezolid, ritonavir)
Dietary supplements (tryptophan)
Antidepressants (trazodone, buspirone)

as a bone"). In the latter group, the patient's mouth is dry ("cotton mouth"), causing a muffled tone. Light responses of the dilated pupil are often absent (because constrictor fibers are inhibited), and many patients are additionally agitated by urinary retention. Commonly identified anticholinergic drugs include diphenhydramine, atropine, and antihistamines, but also many plants such as jimson weed. Treatment is physostigmine (0.5–2.0 mg IV).

Finally, the spectrum of antidepressant intoxication has dramatically changed, and SSRI overdose is now more common. Several other drugs also predispose for serotonin syndrome (Table 10.4).

PERMANENT NEUROTOXICOLOGIC SYMPTOMS

Atypical alcohol ingestion is very problematic and often lethal. Methanol is found in commercial products such as windshield washer fluids, de-icers, antifreeze, paints, wood stains, and glass cleaners. Methanol is metabolized to formaldehyde, and clinical manifestations are delayed for approximately 12–24 hours after ingestion. Marked metabolic acidosis occurs, leading to tachypnea with Kussmaul-type respiration. Neurologic manifestations of atypical alcohol intoxication may also include cranial nerve deficits, ophthalmoplegia, facial palsy, and dysphasia. Similar features are seen at presentation in ethylene glycol intoxication, although the metabolic pathways are different. Tetanic cramps and myoclonus, but also seizures (late in presentation), may occur. In some patients, a markedly increased serum ammonia level and a markedly increased lactate concentration are found, but these could both be spurious with this type of intoxication. This poisoning is difficult to recognize, but if any suspicion exists, an osmolar gap should be sought. The size of the increased osmolar gap also indicates the severity of the intoxication—for example, an osmolar gap of less than 5 mOsmol indicates a smaller ingestion. The osmolar gap is measured as measured osmolality minus calculated osmolality and a correction factor for ingested ethanol should be used if appropriate (mg/dL ÷ 4.6). In later stages after ingestion, the osmolar gap may widen.

Hemodialysis is the only effective treatment for critically ill patients with atypical alcohol ingestion in many hospitals. Triggers to proceed with hemodialysis are the presence of severe metabolic acidosis and decrease in pH and bicarbonate concentration despite bicarbonate therapy, renal failure with creatinine values reaching 2.0 mg/dL, inability to correct an electrolyte imbalance, and a serum methanol level greater than 50 mg/dL. Fomepizole prevents metabolism of methanol (which causes a osmolar gap) into glycolate (which causes an anion gap) and other toxic metabolites; it is a new (albeit expensive) and largely safe addition to treatment of these intoxications. Fomepizole is administered intravenously at 15 mg/kg as a loading dose, followed by a maintenance dose of 10 mg/kg intravenously every 12 hours for 4 doses. One can make a very good argument to immediately start fomepizole (or, if that is unavailable, hemodialysis) in any patient with a suspected intoxication and a marked anion gap acidosis.

Several drugs, if abused, can produce permanent injury. Both amphetamines and cocaine can cause a series of seizures, but also subarachnoid hemorrhage or cerebral hemorrhage if there is a marked hypertensive surge that persists. Some patients also have severe rhabdomyolysis. These patients may get admitted initially with delirium and hallucinations but then become comatose. Any other drug of abuse, such as hallucinogens or barbiturates, can cause respiratory arrest and, through that mechanism, hypoxic-ischemic encephalopathy. An MRI scan is mostly helpful in determining the lesions. Many of these patients have pallidal involvement for the simple reason that it is a watershed area.

Some intoxications can result in seizures (Table 10.5). A major concern is the treatment of seizures in patients who have an overdose with tricyclic antidepressants. These patients present with dilated pupils and continuous myoclonic twitching, and myoclonus should be differentiated from true seizures. Mostly, seizures are seen when the patient has a toxic exposure that has already led to a prolongation of the QRS duration. These patients are at high risk for ventricular arrhythmias and may have to be resuscitated, further confounding the issue of what came first. Treatment of seizures with fosphenytoin loading or use of ketamine or barbiturates for a brief period can control seizures adequately. Additional intravenous sodium bicarbonate is needed in tricyclic antidepressant overdose.

Salicylate overdose can cause neurologic injury through hypoglycemia or cerebral hemorrhages. When salicylates are co-ingested with acetaminophen, marked cerebral edema can occur that needs to be recognized on computed tomography and adequately treated. Hemofiltration dialysis is necessary in many patients.[19,21,22]

Opioid toxicity, mostly from the use of oxycodone for chronic pain management or from heroin injection, can cause permanent injury due to anoxic-ischemic injury. There is a known methadone leukoencephalopathy associated with MRI abnormalities that spare the subcortical U-fibers. Usually, this pattern is seen with methadone intoxication.[17] One case has been reported of an akinetic mutism likely caused by anoxic injury after a methadone overdose.[5] The drugs of abuse can cause significant permanent injury (Table 10.6).

The most concerning intoxication is acetaminophen toxicity.[12] The King's College Hospital with the largest experience in the world has used the ABCD (acidosis, bleeding, creatinine, and drowsiness) mnemonic to diagnose overdose.[9] Acetaminophen overdose immediately causes dramatic damage to the liver, and there is a good

Table 10.5 **Toxins Associated with Seizures**

Organophosphates
Tricyclic antidepressants
Insulin
Sympathomimetics
Cocaine
Amphetamines
Theophylline
Phencyclidine
Ethanol withdrawal
Lithium

From Kunisaki and Augenstein.[10]

correlation between the plasma acetaminophen concentration at a given time after ingestion and development of hepatotoxicity (Figure 10.2). Most intensivists treat when aspartate aminotransferase (AST) levels are elevated, using N-acetylcysteine. (AST levels are increased before abnormal values for prothrombin, international normalized ratio, and bilirubin concentration are evident). Renal failure may follow days later, and patients may need hemodialysis. Fulminant hepatic failure may occur as early as 12 hours after ingestion. Survival in extreme cases is not more than 5%–10%, but liver transplantation improves survival to approximately 70% in 3 years. Patients may rapidly become comatose with worrisome signs such as bilateral extensor posturing, but brainstem reflexes should remain normal for patients to survive the ordeal.

Table 10.6 **Major Consequences of Common Drugs of Abuse**

Class	Neurologic manifestations	Late concerns
Amphetamines	Mydriasis, paranoia, hallucinations, delirium, focal signs (cerebral hemorrhage)	Cerebral infarcts (vasculopathy)
Cocaine	Seizures (complex partial type) and dystonia, chorea, migraine, coma (subarachnoid hemorrhage), rhabdomyolysis	Transient ischemic attack, cerebral infarction, aneurysmal rupture
Barbiturates	Coma, hypoxic-ischemic encephalopathy (shock), respiratory arrest	Persistent vegetative state, cerebral infarct
Hallucinogens	Colored geometric images, catalepsy, mydriasis, piloerection, insomnia, hyperthermia, coma	Ischemic stroke, cognitive decline

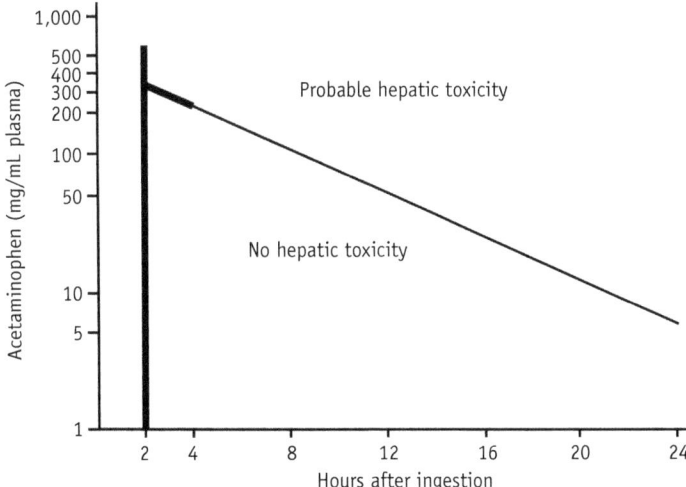

Figure 10.2 Ingestion of acetaminophen and risk of liver injury (Example of the Rumack-Matthew nomogram). (From Rumack BH.[17])

In these patients, the initial symptomatology is hepatic encephalopathy, but this rapidly transitions to a structural injury that involves diffuse brain edema and increased intracranial pressure (ICP). The injury can be immediately severe with a rapid loss of brainstem reflexes, and the patient may become brain dead within a matter of hours. This can all occur despite ICP monitor placement and a serious attempt to reduce increased ICP. Patients who in addition have progressive coagulopathy are at increased risk for intracranial hemorrhages, although these are rarely seen (and if they are, they are related to placement of the ICP monitor). Further management of brain edema has been discussed in Chapter 4.[3,4,14]

Cases of survival after intentional carbon monoxide intoxication are rarely seen. The earliest signs of carbon monoxide poisoning are personality changes, including loss of orderliness, snapping at people, and outbursts of anxiety, but also profound headache and diminished responsiveness when the carboxyhemoglobin concentration increases. The classic cherry-red coloration of the skin is not common, and because of tissue hypoxia, patients are more likely to be cyanotic. Severe papilledema with peripapillary flame hemorrhages may occur and could be a direct result of asphyxia. Carbon monoxide binds to hemoglobin with a great affinity, resulting in the compound carboxyhemoglobin and effectively reducing the capacity of hemoglobin to carry oxygen to tissue. However, the bond of carbon monoxide to the heme group remains reversible and is released by high concentrations of oxygen. Additional significant effects are a leftward shift in the oxyhemoglobin dissociation curve, particularly at concentrations greater than 50%, which reduces oxygen release from remaining oxyhemoglobin. Acute leukoencephalopathy and necrosis of the globus pallidus is often seen on CT or MRI and is present in comatose patients, and also predicts poor outcome. Treatment of acute carbon monoxide poisoning is 100% high-flow oxygen and, if that is unsuccessful, hyperbaric oxygen.

Then there are inhalants. The so-called volatile substance abuse problem includes products such as aerosols and dry cleaner fluids, some of which contain ingredients that damage the brain. Injury may also be related to suffocation from plastic bags or as a result of vomit. The acute effects of inhalants include hallucinations, sometimes in the setting of a full psychotic break. In exceptional cases, acute effects involve acute leukoencephalopathy.

Putting It All Together

- Suicide and illicit drug use are the main causes of intoxication in the ICU.
- ICU mortality in patients with serious intoxication is low.
- ICU mortality is high in persistently comatose patients with structural injury.
- Patients with intoxication from atypical alcohols or acetaminophen require more aggressive and complex care that may include permanent dialysis or liver transplantation.

References

1. Brandenburg R, Brinkman S, de Keizer NF, Meulenbelt J, de Lange DW. In-hospital mortality and long-term survival of patients with acute intoxication admitted to the ICU. *Crit Care Med* 2014;42:1471–1479.
2. Clark BJ, Binswanger IA, Moss M. The intoxicated ICU patient: another opportunity to improve long-term outcomes. *Crit Care Med* 2014;42:1563–1564.
3. Dargan PI, Jones AL. Acetaminophen poisoning: an update for the intensivist. *Crit Care* 2002;6:108–110.
4. Dargan PI, Jones AL. Management of paracetamol poisoning. *Trends Pharmacol Sci* 2003; 24:154–157.
5. Gheuens S, Michotte A, Flamez A, De Keyser J. Delayed akinetic catatonic mutism following methadone overdose. *Neurotoxicology* 2010;31:762–764.
6. Henderson A, Wright M, Pond SM. Experience with 732 acute overdose patients admitted to an intensive care unit over six years. *Med J Aust* 1993;158:28–30.
7. Heyerdahl F, Bjornas MA, Hovda KE, et al. Acute poisonings treated in hospitals in Oslo—a one-year prospective study (II): clinical outcome. *Clin Toxicol* 2008;46:42–49.
8. Heyerdahl F, Hovda KE, Bjornaas MA, et al. Clinical assessment compared to laboratory screening in acutely poisoned patients. *Hum Exp Toxicol* 2008;27:73–79.
9. Kelham MD, Goundry AL. ABCD: a simple mnemonic for the King's College Hospital criteria in paracetamol overdose. *Br J Hosp Med* 2014;75:716.
10. Kunisaki TA, Augenstein WL. Drug- and toxin-induced seizures. *Emerg Med Clin North Am* 1994;12:1027–1056.
11. Lam SM, Lau AC, Yan WW. Over 8 years experience on severe acute poisoning requiring intensive care in Hong Kong, China. *Hum Exp Toxicol* 2010;29:757–765.
12. Lancaster EM, Hiatt JR, Zarrinpar A. Acetaminophen hepatotoxicity: an updated review. *Arch Toxicol*. 2015;89:193–199.
13. Menghini VV, Albright RC Jr. Treatment of lithium intoxication with continuous venovenous hemodiafiltration. *Am J Kidney Dis* 2000;36:E21.

14. Mohsenin V. Assessment and management of cerebral edema and intracranial hypertension in acute liver failure. *J Crit Care* 2013;28:783–791.
15. Nelson LS, Lewin NA, Howland MA, et al., eds. *Goldfrank's Toxicologic Emergencies*. 9th ed. New York: McGraw-Hill, 2011.
16. Pedavally S, Fugate JE, Rabinstein AA. Serotonin syndrome in the intensive care unit: clinical presentations and precipitating medications. *Neurocrit Care* 2014;21:108–113.
17. Rumack BH: Acetaminophen hepatotoxicity: the first 35 years. *J Toxicol Clin Toxicol* 2002;40:3–20.
18. Rusyniak DE, Sprague JE. Toxin-induced hyperthermic syndromes. *Med Clin North Am* 2005;89:1277–1296.
19. Salgado RA, Jorens PG, Baar I, et al. Methadone-induced toxic leukoencephalopathy: MR imaging and MR proton spectroscopy findings. *Am J Neuroradiol* 2010;31:565–566.
20. Scharman EJ. Methods used to decrease lithium absorption or enhance elimination. *J Toxicol Clin Toxicol* 1997;35:601–608.
21. Thisted B, Krantz T, Stroom J, Sorensen MB. Acute salicylate self-poisoning in 177 consecutive patients treated in ICU. *Acta Anaesthesiol Scand* 1987;31:312–316.
22. Timmer RT, Sands JM. Lithium intoxication. *J Am Soc Nephrol* 1999;10:666–674.
23. Wood DM, Dargan PI, Jones AL. Measuring plasma salicylate concentrations in all patients with drug overdose or altered consciousness: is it necessary? *Emerg Med J* 2005;22:401–403.
24. Wrathall G, Sinclair R, Moore A, Pogson D. Three case reports of the use of hemodiafiltration in the treatment of salicylate overdose. *Hum Exp Toxicol* 2001;20:491–495.

Index

ABCD. *See* acidosis, bleeding, creatinine, and drowsiness mnemonic
abulia, 22, 26*t*
acetaminophen, 145–46, 147*f*
acetylcholine, 6, 18, 18*t*
acidosis, bleeding, creatinine, and drowsiness (ABCD) mnemonic, 145–46
acquired weakness
  conclusions, 101–3
  critical illness polyneuropathy and, 94, 96*f*
  defined, 99
  electrophysiologic study, 101
  evaluation, 99–100, 99*f*, 102
  examination for, 94
  flaccid quadriparesis and, 99–100
  immobilization and, 98–99
  inflammation and, 96
  MUSCLES mnemonic and, 99, 99*f*
  neuromuscular blocking agents and, 96–98, 98*f*
  neuromuscular conditions causing, 95*t*
  nutrition and, 98, 102
  overview, 93–94
  phrenic nerve injury and, 102
  polyneuropathy and myopathy mechanisms and, 96, 97*f*
  in practice, 99–103
  principles, 94–99
  rhabdomyolysis and, 99
action myoclonus, 83*t*
acute adrenal disease, 39–40
acute cauda equina syndrome, 66
acute confusion
  CAM-ICU and, 21, 22*t*, 23*t*, 24–25*t*, 24*t*
  classification of, 19–26
  conclusions about, 30
  lab tests, 27
  mechanisms, 18–19
  neurologic findings, 21, 22, 26*t*
  neurotransmitters and, 18, 18*t*
  overview, 17
  in practice, 26–30
  principles, 18–25

  risk factors, 26–27, 27*f*
  sedative agents and, 18–19
  symptoms, 18
  terminology surrounding, 20
  treatment of, 27–30, 28*t*, 29*t*
acute hemiparesis, 13
acute in-stent thrombosis, 70–71
acute liver failure, 36–38, 38*f*
acute metabolic derangements, 125–26
acute pancreatic disease, 38
Acute Physiology and Chronic Health Evaluation (APACHE), 139*t*
acute pulmonary disease, 34
acute renal failure, 34–36
acute subdural hematoma, 115–16
acute thyroid failure, 39
ADC. *See* apparent diffusion coefficient
Addison's disease. *See* acute adrenal disease
α-adrenergic agonists, 140*t*
agitated patients, 21*f*
agnosia, 26, 26*t*
α_2-agonists, 19
ALS. *See* amyotrophic lateral sclerosis
American Spinal Injury Association scale, 110
ammonia, 36–37
amphetamines, 142, 145, 146*t*
amyotrophic lateral sclerosis (ALS), 10, 94
aneurysms, 64, 64*f*, 65, 72, 113
anoxic-ischemic injury, to brain, 79, 79*f*, 83*t*
anterior horn cell disorders, 95*t*
anterior interosseous nerve, 113
anterior spinal artery, 62
anticoagulation, 11
antiepileptics, 11, 141*t*
antipsychotics, 141*t*
aortic disease, 65–66
APACHE. *See* Acute Physiology and Chronic Health Evaluation
aphasia, 22, 26, 26*t*
apoptosis, 79*f*
apparent diffusion coefficient (ADC), 86, 86*f*
atrial fibrillation, 52–53

151

INDEX

autonomic storming, 10
axillary nerve damage, 114

barbiturates, 139f, 143, 146t
benzodiazepines, 5, 54–55, 139f, 142, 143
bevacizumab, 128t
β-blockers, 141t
blood pressure fluctuation, in spinal cord injury, 11
blunt vascular trauma, 110, 112t
bortezomib, 124
brachial plexopathy, 48t
brachial plexus, 114, 117
brain injury. *See also* traumatic brain injury
   anoxic-ischemic, 79, 79f, 83t
   conclusions, 88–89
   hypothermia and, 80–81
   imaging and, 87, 86f
   overview, 77–78
   principles, 78–83
   prognosis, 78, 84–88
   questions regarding, 77–78
brain metastases, 128, 129
brainstem, 83, 86, 88, 131t
Brown-Sequard syndrome, 66
buspirone, 144t
busulfan, 124

CABG. *See* coronary artery bypass graft
cachexia, 96
calcium channel blockers, 141t, 142
CAM-ICU. *See* Confusion Assessment Method for the Intensive Care Unit
cancer. *See* neurooncologic emergencies
capecitabine, 128t
carbon monoxide, 140t, 147
cardiac arrest
   American Academy of Neurology guidelines regarding, 84–85
   conclusions, 88–89
   CPR and, 77
   hypothermia and, 81
   LINC and, 80, 80f
   overview, 77–78
   postresuscitation disease and, 81
   in practice, 84–88
   principles, 78–83
   prognosis, 84–88
   questions regarding, 77–78
   TTM and, 84, 84t
cardiac patient, postoperative
   atrial fibrillation and, 52–53
   CABG and, 47, 49–51, 49f, 52t
   coma and, 54
   complications, 58
   complications mechanisms in, 48t
   conclusions, 57–58
   infectious endocarditis and, 55
   nerve injury, 56
   neuroimaging and, 51–52
   overview, 47–48
   in practice, 53–56
   principles, 48–52
   seizures and, 54–55
   stroke and, 52, 53f, 55
cardiopulmonary resuscitation (CPR)
   ECMO and, 82–83
   limits of, 79
   LINC and, 80, 80f
   mortality and, 77
carotid disease, 66–67
   hypotension and, 69, 70t
   stenting and, 69, 69f
carotid endarterectomy, 71
carotid revascularization, 61, 67
Carotid Revascularization Endarterectomy Versus Stenting Trial (CREST), 67
central nervous system (CNS)
   infections, in cancer, 132
   neurooncologic emergencies and, 123, 123f, 124f, 132
   primary lymphoma of, 129–30, 129f
central spinal fluid (CSF), 68, 68t
cerebellar degeneration, 131t
cerebral blood flow, 34, 35f
cerebral edema, 37
cerebral hyperperfusion syndrome, 67, 70–71
cerebral vessels injury, 116
cerebrospinal pressure (CSF), 62
cervical spine
   curbside consultations and, 10
   stroke and, 110
chemotherapy-associated complications, 124
chemotherapy drugs, 126–27, 127t
CIP. *See* critical illness polyneuromyopathy; critical illness polyneuropathy
cisplatin, 126t
cisplatinum, 124
clonidine, 18t, 141t
CMAPs. *See* compound muscle action potentials
CNS. *See* central nervous system
cocaine, 145, 146t
coma
   cardiac patient, postoperative, and, 53–54
   CPR and, 77
   hypothermia and, 80–81
   prognosis and, 78
   statistics, 88
compound muscle action potentials (CMAPs), 101
computed tomography (CT), 8–9
Confusion Assessment Method for the Intensive Care Unit (CAM-ICU), 21, 22t, 23t, 24–25t, 24t
consultation. *See also* curbside consultation; *specific topic*
   assessment approach, 13–14
   benefits, 12, 12f
   cause of illness and, 6
   conclusions about, 15
   considerations, general, 3
   drugs and, 5–6, 5t
   essentials, 14t

family discussions and, 7
issues surrounding, 1–3
phone calls and, 2
in practice, 7–15
principles, 3–7
reasons for, 4t, 13
therapeutic hypothermia and, 6
timeliness of, 4–5
corneal reflex, 87t
coronary artery bypass graft (CABG), 47, 49–51, 49f, 52t
corticosteroids, 97
CPR. *See* cardiopulmonary resuscitation
Crawford classification, of thoracoabdominal aneurysms, 64, 64f, 65
CREST. *See* Carotid Revascularization Endarterectomy Versus Stenting Trial
critical illness polyneuromyopathy (CIP), 93
cachexia and, 96
electrophysiology and, 100
management of, 102
mechanisms of injury, 96, 97f
critical illness polyneuropathy (CIP), 93
acquired weakness and, 94, 96, 96f, 97f
blood glucose and, 94
electrophysiology and, 100
management of, 102
mechanisms of injury, 96, 97f
statistics, 103
CSF. *See* central spinal fluid; cerebrospinal pressure
CT. *See* computed tomography
curbside consultation
anticoagulation and, 11
antiepileptics and, 11
autonomic storming and, 10
avoidance of, 2
blood pressure fluctuation and, 10
cervical spine clearance, 10
common questions, 8–11
CT scans and, 7–8
defined, 3
determining need for, 3–4
EEG interpretation, 8–9
issues surrounding, 4
Parkinson's disease and, 11
ventilator weaning and, 9–10
when to deliver, 8f
Cushing's syndrome, 126
cyclophosphamide, 126t

delayed cognitive dysfunction, 48t
delirium, 20. *See also* acute confusion
Denver criteria, 111, 112t
depolarizing blockers, 97
depolarizing muscle relaxants, 6
dermatomyositis, 100
Determining Neurologic Outcomes from Valve Operations Study, 47
dexmedetomidine, 5t, 18t

dialysis, 36
diaphragmatic atrophy, 9
dieback, 124
diffusion-weighted imaging (DWI), 87, 86f
donepezil, 18t
dopamine, 18, 18t
drugs. *See also* neurotoxicology
chemotherapy, 126–27, 127t
consultation and, 5–6, 5t
DWI. *See* diffusion-weighted imaging
dystonia, 13

ECMO. *See* extracorporeal membrane oxygenation
electroencephalography (EEG), 8–9
electromyography (EMG), 9
encephalomyelitis, 131t
encephalopathy, 20, 48t
ethanol, 139f, 140t, 143, 146t
excitotoxicity, 79f
extracorporeal membrane oxygenation (ECMO), 77
device, 82f
postresuscitation disease and, 81–82, 82f
survival rate and, 82–83

fat embolization syndrome, 113, 113t, 116–17, 116f
fentanyl, 141t
clearance, 5, 5t
dosage, 5
flaccid quadriparesis, 99–100
flumazenil, 37, 143
fomepizole, 145
FOUR. *See* Full Outline of UnResponsiveness Score
fractures, 109
Full Outline of UnResponsiveness (FOUR) Score, 41

gabapentin, 10
gefitinib, 128t
glucocorticoids, 97
Gurd's criteria, 113t

hallucinogens, 146t
haloperidol, 18t, 28
hangman's fracture, 109
Hashimoto's encephalopathy, 39
hematologic malignancies, 122
hemorrhagic stroke, 48t
hepatic encephalopathy
ICP monitor and, 43, 43f
MARS and, 41–42, 42f
stages, 41, 42t
treatment of, 41–43
heroin, 142
Horner's syndrome, 48t, 114
hyperactive delirium, 20
hypercalcemia, 125
hypercarbia, 41
hypercoagulability, 35
hypertonic saline, 115
hypoglycemic, 125

hypoglycemics, 140t
hypotension, 69, 70t
hypothermia, therapeutic, 6
  coma and, 81
  criticisms of, 87–88
  meta-analysis regarding, 87–88, 87t
  overview, 78
  reflexes and, 85
hypoxemia, 34
hypoxic-ischemic encephalopathy (HIE), 48t

IABP. *See* intraaortic balloon pump
ICP. *See* intracranial pressure monitor
idiogenic osmole hypothesis, 36
ifosfamide, 124
immobilization, 98–99
infectious endocarditis, 55
inflammation, 40, 96
inhalants, 148
insulin, 146t
intercostal arteries, 62
intoxications symptoms, 139f
intraaortic balloon pump (IABP), 56, 57
intracranial pressure (ICP) monitor
  hepatic encephalopathy and, 43, 43f
  managing, 109
  Marshall's classification and, 108–9, 109t
ischemic infarction, 48t

ketamine, 18t

Lambert-Eaton myasthenic syndrome, 100
lapatinib, 128t
leptomeningeal carcinomatosis, 124f
leptomeningeal metastasis, 128, 128t
levetiracetam, 55
limbic, brainstem, hypothalamic encephalitis, 131t
linezolid, 144t
lipopolysaccharide (LPS), 40
liposomal cytarabine, 128t
lithium, 139f, 141t, 143, 146t
lorazepam, 5t, 29t
LPS. *See* lipopolysaccharide
LUCAS in Cardiac Arrest, 80, 80f
lumbosacral plexus, 115

magnetic resonance imaging (MRI), 87, 86f
man-in-the-barrel syndrome, 83t
mannitol, 115
MARS. *See* Molecular Adsorbent Recirculating System
Marshall's classification, 108–9, 109t
median nerve injury, 114
Medical Research Council (MRC) sum score, 99
melatonin, 18, 18t
Memphis criteria, 111, 112t
methanol and ethylene glycol, 141t, 144–45
methotrexate, 124, 128t
metoclopramide, 144t
midazolam, 5t, 29t

midodrine, 69
Molecular Adsorbent Recirculating System (MARS), 42–43, 42f
motor score, 87t
motor unit potentials, 101
MRC. *See* Medical Research Council sum score
MRI. *See* magnetic resonance imaging
multiorgan failure, 40
muscle
  CMAPs, 101
  diseases, 95t
  relaxants, 6
MUSCLES mnemonic, 99, 99f
myoclonic jerks, 9
myoclonic status epilepticus, 87t
myoclonus, 13
myopathies, 100

NAIM. *See* nonvasculitic autoimmune meningoencephalitis
NCSE. *See* nonconvulsive status epilepticus
nerve injury, 48t, 56, 102, 113
neuroleptics, 140t
neuromuscular blocking agents, 96–98, 98f
neuromuscular junction (NMJ), 94, 95t, 100
neuron-specific enolase (NSE), 85, 87t
neurooncologic emergencies
  acute metabolic derangements and, 125–26
  brain metastases, 128, 129
  chemotherapy-associated complications, 124
  CNS and, 123, 123f, 124f, 132
  CNS infections in, 132
  conclusions, 132–33
  hematologic malignancies and, 122
  hypercalcemia, 125
  hypoglycemic, 125
  leptomeningeal metastasis and, 128, 128t
  overview, 121–22
  pain and, 127
  paraneoplastic endocrinopathies, 125
  paraneoplastic syndromes, 130, 131t
  patient mix and, 122–23
  in practice, 126–32
  presenting semiology of, 126–27, 126t
  primary CNS lymphoma, 129, 129f, 130
  principles, 122–26
  statistics, 133
  stroke and, 130–32
  tumor lysis syndrome, 25
  ventilation and, 122
neurotoxicology
  APACHE categorization, 139t
  common intoxications symptoms, 139f
  conclusions, 148
  mechanisms of, 142
  overdosed patient and, 138–42
  overview, 137–38
  permanent symptoms, 144–48
  principles of, 142–48

screening, 141, 141*t*
seizures and, 145, 146*t*
serotonin syndrome, 144, 144*t*
transient symptoms, 143–44
neurotransmitters, acute confusion and, 18, 18*t*
NMDA. *See N*-methyl-D-aspartate
N-methyl-D-aspartate (NMDA), 18, 18*t*
NMJ. *See* neuromuscular junction
nonconvulsive status epilepticus (NCSE), 2, 9
non-depolarizing blockers, 97
nondepolarizing muscle relaxants, 6
nonvasculitic autoimmune meningoencephalitis (NAIM), 39
noradrenaline, 18, 18*t*
NSE. *See* neuron-specific enolase
nutrition, 98, 102

olanzapine, 18*t*
ondansetron, 144*t*
opioids, 145
opsoclonus myoclonus syndrome, 131*t*
Oral Trail Making Test, 22
organ disfunction
   acute adrenal disease, 39–40
   acute liver failure, 36–38, 38*f*
   acute pancreatic disease, 38
   acute pulmonary disease, 34
   acute renal failure, 34–36
   acute thyroid failure, 38–39
   conclusions, 44
   multiorgan failure, 40
   overview, 33
   in practice, 41–43
   principles, 33–42
organophosphates, 146*t*
overdosed patient, 138–42
oxaliplatin, 124
oxcarbazepine, 126*t*
oxycodone, 145

paclitaxel, 124
pain, 127
paraneoplastic endocrinopathies, 125
paraneoplastic syndromes, 130, 131*t*
paraplegia, 67–68
Parkinsonism, 83*t*
Parkinson's disease, 11
PEEP. *See* positive end-expiratory pressure
perioperative myocardial infarction,
perioperative stroke, 70
peripheral nerves damage, 114
peripheral neuropathies, 95*t*
phencyclidine, 146*t*
phenylephrine, 69
phrenic nerve injury, 48*t*, 102
pituitary apoplexy, 48*t*
polyneuropathy, 10. *See also* critical illness polyneuropathy
polytrauma
   acute subdural hematoma and, 115–16

aneurysms and, 113
brachial plexus and, 114, 117
cerebral vessels injury and, 116
conclusions, 117
examination, 115
fat embolism syndrome and, 113, 113*t*, 116–17, 116*f*
instability and, 108
lumbosacral plexus and, 113–14
Marshall's classification and, 108–9, 109*t*
overview, 107
peripheral nerves and, 114
posterior fossa and, 108
in practice, 115–17
principles, 108–14
spinal cord and, 109–10, 117
statistics, 117
stroke and, 110, 112*t*
vertebral artery injury and, 110*f*, 111*f*, 116
positive end-expiratory pressure (PEEP), 113, 115
posterior fossa, 108
posterior reversible encephalopathy syndrome (PRES), 33, 35–36, 124
posterior spinal artery, 62
postresuscitation disease, 81, 82*f*
PRES. *See* posterior reversible encephalopathy syndrome
primary CNS lymphoma, 129, 129*f*, 130
propofol, 5*t*, 18*t*, 29*t*
pupillary reflex, 87*t*

quetiapine, 18*t*
quiet delirium, 20

radial nerve paralysis, 114
reflexes, 85
reperfusion, 79
restenosis, 67
reverse urea hypothesis, 36
rhabdomyolysis, 99
ritonavir, 144*t*
rituximab, 128*t*
rivastigmine, 18*t*

salicylates, 140*t*, 145
saphenous nerve, 57
sciatic nerve damage, 114
sedative agents, 140*t*
   acute confusion and, 18–19
seizures, 48*t*
   cardiac patient, postoperative, and, 54–55
   chemotherapy drugs and, 126–27, 127*t*
   neurotoxicology and, 145, 146*t*
sepsis, 40
serotonin, 18, 18*t*
   reuptake inhibitors, 141*t*
   syndrome, 144, 144*t*
SIADH. *See* syndrome of inappropriate antidiuretic hormone

SIRS. *See* systemic inflammatory reaction syndrome
small-cell lung cancer (SCLC), 125–26
solvents, 141*t*
somatosensory-evoked potential, 87*t*
spinal cord
  American Spinal Injury Association scale and, 110
  blood pressure fluctuation and, 11
  blood supply, 62–65, 63*f*, 64*f*
  brachial plexus injury and, 117
  disorders, 95*t*
  evaluation of, 109–10
  fractures and, 109
  leptomeningeal carcinomatosis and, 124*f*
  paraplegia and, 67–68
spinal cord ischemia (SCI), 56, 61
  clamping and, 65
  management, 68–69, 68*t*
  vascular surgery and, 72
starfield pattern, 113
stenting, 67, 67*t*, 69*f*
steroid-responsive encephalopathy associated with autoimmune thyroiditis (SREAT), 39
stiff-man syndrome, 131*t*
stroke
  blunt vascular trauma and, 110, 112*t*
  cardiac patient, postoperative, and, 52, 53*f*, 55
  hemorrhagic, 48*t*
  neurooncologic emergencies and, 130–32
  perioperative, 67*t*, 69–70
strychnine, 141*t*
subacute sensory neuronopathy, 131*t*
subclavian steal syndrome, 48*t*
subsyndromal delirium, 20
succinylcholine, 6, 98*f*
sulcal artery, 62
sumatriptan, 144*t*
sympathetic hyperactivity syndrome. *See* autonomic storming
sympathicomimetics, 140, 140*t*
sympathomimetics, 146*t*
syncope, 9
syndrome of inappropriate antidiuretic hormone (SIADH), 125
systemic inflammatory reaction syndrome (SIRS), 40

TAA. *See* thoracic aortic aneurysm
Targeted Temperature Management After Cardiac Arrest (TTM), 84, 84*t*
TBI. *See* traumatic brain injury
TEE. *See* transesophageal echocardiography
TEVAR. *See* thoracic endovascular aortic repair
theophylline, 146*t*
thoracic aortic aneurysm (TAA), 72
thoracic endovascular aortic repair (TEVAR), 72
transesophageal echocardiography (TEE), 11
traumatic brain injury (TBI)
  acute subdural hematoma and, 115–16
  aneurysms and, 113
  cerebral vessels injury and, 116
  conclusions, 117
  instability and, 108
  Marshall's classification and, 108–9, 109*t*
  overview, 107
  posterior fossa and, 108
  vertebral artery injury and, 110*f*, 111*f*, 116
trazodone, 144*t*
tricyclic antidepressants, 146*t*
tryptophan, 144*t*
tumor lysis syndrome, 25

uremic retention solutes, 34–35

valproate, 55, 144*t*
valve surgery, 47
varicella zoster virus (VZV), 132
vascular surgery, postoperative
  aortic disease, 65–66
  carotid disease, 66–67
  cerebrospinal pressure and, 62
  complications, 72
  conclusions, 71–72
  Crawford classification and, 64, 64*f*, 65
  overview, 61
  paraplegia and, 67–68
  in practice, 67–71
  principles, 62–67
  SCI and, 68, 68*t*, 72
  spinal cord blood supply and, 62–65, 63*f*, 64*f*
vasculitic neuropathy, 100
vecuronium, 5*t*, 98*f*
ventilation
  neurooncologic emergencies and, 122
  weaning from, 9–10
vertebral artery injury, 110, 111*f*, 116
vincristine, 124
visual loss, 48*t*
VZV. *See* varicella zoster virus

weakness. *See* acquired weakness
withdrawal of active care, 84*t*

www.ingramcontent.com/pod-product-compliance
Ingram Content Group UK Ltd.
Pitfield, Milton Keynes, MK11 3LW, UK
UKHW021255180426
11947UKWH00010B/785